Un-Glued

Un-Glued

THE SECRET SCIENCE OF STEM CELLS
THAT DISSOLVE THE EFFECTS OF SUGAR

Dr. Richard P. Jacoby, DPM
Past President of the Association of Extremity Nerve Surgeons

Dr. Richard Jacoby
drjacobybook@gmail.com

ISBN: 979-8-9909863-1-2 (paperback)
ISBN: 979-8-9909863-2-9 (ebook)
ISBN: 979-8-9909863-0-5 (hardcover)

Ordering Information:
Special discounts are available on quantity purchases by corporations, associations, and others. For details, email drjacobybook@gmail.com.

Table of Contents

Prologue

Good health can seem complicated and fraught with multiple diagnoses, not unlike coming upon a tragic automobile accident. At first glance, all that can be seen are the pieces strewn about—individual shards of glass, crushed metal, or mangled bodies—but the cause of the crash appears to be a mystery. How did the tragedy happen? What would have prevented such carnage?

Lots of wonderful, laudable books about good health have failed to identify the underlying root cause of disease. Gary Taubes's book *Rethinking Diabetes: What Science Reveals About Diet, Insulin, and Successful Treatments*; Richard Johnson's book *Nature Wants Us to Be Fat: The Surprising Science Behind Why We Gain Weight and How We Can Prevent—and Reverse—It*; and even Peter Attia's most recent book, *Outlive: The Science and Art of Longevity.*

In fact, my greatest criticism of all the books I've read on the subject of sugar, in general or about a specific disease like diabetes, is that none of the authors see it from my perspective—the lens of a simple podiatric surgeon trying to solve the challenge of an inflamed nerve. As you will see in the following chapters, the understanding has nothing to do with intelligence and everything to do with viewpoint.

Viewpoint, in fact, is crucial. The wonderful children's guessing game of "can you see what I see?" asks one to look through another's lens. The game's simple question is the crux of all arguments, from political to philosophical. The only answer is no. *One* cannot until they look through *another's* lens. Like radio waves, the object may be invisible without "the right lens." Nevertheless, the truth is still there. Looking through another's lens is when epiphanies happen.

The visible truth is what my mentor, A. Lee Dellon, MD, PhD, with Johns Hopkins University at the time, showed me in the late 1990s: The chemistry of sugar causes inflammation and physical compression of a specific nerve; that was Dellon's conclusion for the pain and suffering he was finding in patients with debilitating carpal tunnel syndrome. When I joined him in his surgery, literally looking through his magnification lens, I could suddenly *see* the connection between sugar to every other type of nerve in the body. My conclusion was that sugar (especially carbohydrates found in all processed foods) is poisoning us.

In my first book, *Sugar Crush* (2015), I established the scientific groundwork for my theory of global compression, which explains how sugar leads to the destruction of nerves throughout the body. In the following excerpt, I revealed how sugar *initiates and exacerbates* sugar-induced illness like diabetic ulcers, Morton's neuroma, and much, much worse.

> Bite after bite, sip after sip, sugar is inflaming your blood vessels and nerves. This unrelenting inflammation incites stress

in the body's natural repair system, which results in *fibrosis* (scarring). The ongoing scarring systematically, pervasively, and insidiously causes compression in any area where blood vessels and nerves pass together through a tight area.

The Global Compression Theory
Sugar (glucose) = Chronic Inflammation +
Trauma (compression or injury) =
Nerve Damage, Pain, and Dysfunction

- Excess glucose (the sugar found in all carbohydrates) causes chronic inflammation within the nerves. This result causes their normally smooth surfaces to become sticky—catching and accumulating all kinds of micro-scopic particles.[1]

  This effect was vividly described by friend and colleague John Cooke, MD, PhD, who believes inflammatory substances like sugar also cause the inner lining of arteries to become less like Teflon and more like Velcro.
- In turn, the nerves passing through narrow tunnels within bones and ligaments are slowly compressed—squeezed shut and crushed.
- Add trauma (such as repetitive motion), and you have nerve damage, pain, and dysfunction.

This simple truth extends to *every* peripheral nerve, not only those exhibiting as carpal tunnel in the hands or tarsal tunnel in the feet. In fact, my clinical experience convinces me that while the tsunami of disease we are experiencing is affected by numerous universal forces, many diseases we think of as separate and distinct

---

1   The inflammation and accumulated sticky gunk cause the scarring called fibrosis.

are instead end-stage manifestations of the same flawed process from excess sugar consumption, resulting in global compression.

It's not multiple diseases, but rather a single mechanism that's making us sick. Various names have been given to these areas of compression, leading to the *false* idea that amyotrophic lateral sclerosis (also known as ALS or Lou Gehrig's disease), autism, Parkinson's, Alzheimer's, multiple sclerosis, and other so-called autoimmune diseases such as rheumatoid arthritis—and even cancer—are separate and distinct diseases. In fact, they all are compression neuropathies with separate names given to them centuries ago. All are manifestations of "sugar poisoning"—an excess of refined sugars and processed foods.[2] The goal of *Un-Glued* is to present the details of my thesis—as well as to illustrate ways in which foods are being rammed down our throats by the greed of big business and sloppy governance from those charged with protecting us.

I'm gratified that many other professionals in the medical field (including popular health influencers such as David Perlmutter, MD, Thomas Seyfried, PhD, Joseph Mercola, DO) now fully embrace this concept and that emerging research and new discoveries in biochemistry continue to bolster my theories.

Now, with *Un-Glued* I explore:

- How through the technology of electron microscopy, we can see the gossamer-like filaments of **glu**cose (literally

---

2   It's key to note the phrase "processed foods" because most contain high levels of wheat, corn, potatoes, rice, fruit, and processed sugars (yes, even organic), all of which the body chemically converts to glucose—a.k.a., blood sugar. More in later chapters on the chemistry of how this occurs.

sticky sugar) that hold our cells together as they fortify at-risk cells and fend off invaders.

- How *too much* **glu**cose is still the genesis of disease—and how the primary defense against disease and inflammation is to become ***un*-glued.**

- Increasing evidence that cancer is a metabolic disease—and that **glu**cose and **glu**tamine (an amino acid often taken as a weight-loss, body-building supplement) feed it. Therefore, we should be starving cancer of sugar, not poisoning it and us with radiation and chemo.

- How through the science of epigenetics, food can alter the way the body *interprets* DNA sequencing. The consequence means that you not only pass along eating behaviors to your children, but you also can pass along reactions to food toxins that then manifest as disease.

- New evidence that *sugar plus stress*—not the old whipping boy, saturated fat—is the leading cause of arterial plaque (sticky gunk turned hard, a.k.a., atherosclerosis).

- Increased sugar intake is a major risk factor for dementia.

- How the global compression theory explains tragic and explosive increases in autism.

- How stem cell therapies can temporarily mitigate the pain and past damage of sugar and why, despite being extremely simple to execute, it's so damned expensive to procure.

- How the high-fructose corn syrup (super sugar found in processed foods) blocks leptin—the hormonal switch that normally tells you that you've had enough to eat, that you are satisfied and satiated.

- How to beat sugar addiction once and for all.

Most importantly, I want to convince you that by taking charge of what you eat, you can not only prevent but also immediately begin reversing these devastating effects that sugar is having on your body and your overall health.

You can *un*-glue yourself!

NOT JUST ANOTHER CATCHY BOOK TITLE

I'm sure catchy book titles sell more books, but creating a clever title was not my main purpose in choosing the title for this book.

How did I come up with the title *Un-Glued*? I was at a think tank in California when I first used the word, and somebody asked me what it meant. I gave him the answer in the language of chemistry.

"No, no," he said. "What's the *word* mean?"

That prompted me to look up the history of the word *glucose* that had become so critical to my professional and personal goals. Turns out it was coined in 1840 by French chemist Eugène Melchior Péligot, taken from the ancient Greek, *gleukos* "sweet wine" (related to *glykos* "sweet") and the Latin suffix "-ose" meaning "full of" or "abounding in."[3] As he was studying sugar at the time, biochemists came to designate all sugars with the suffix "-ose." Much more on that later.

The true purpose of this book is not to give you a history lesson or have you brush up on medical terminology. My intent is to

---

3   And since Péligot was French, it's easy to surmise that he may have also associated the sticky substance to the Latin word for glue, *gluten,* as well as the Old French word for glue, *glu.*

show you that you are not suffering because of a thousand and one different diseases—you're suffering only from *one* because of the harmful effects of sugar.

The good news is that you can become *un*-glued. Becoming *un*-glued simply means undoing a lifetime of damage caused by the sticky, sweet substance glued to the walls of your veins and arteries, clogging them and obstructing your nerves. The harder way to do it is to remove all sugar from your diet and facilitate the body's natural healing mechanisms. The easier way is the glory of stem cells, which speed up that process and allow you to experience the benefits of healing almost immediately—albeit not long-lasting if you continue to consume excess sugar.

THE "DO I EVEN NEED THIS BOOK?" QUIZ

Don't worry; it's short and painless. Just check every true statement.

_____ I believe exercise fixes overeating. *Calories in/calories out.*

_____ I'm the one who refills the office candy bowl and surprises my team with donuts.

_____ I know that animal fat is bad for me.

_____ I have *two* pill-organizers, one for breakfast and one for bedtime.

_____ I consume alcohol at social gatherings. Okay, at least once a day.

_____ If I stop at a fast-food place, I know what I want without looking at the menu.

_____ I've had something precancerous removed.

_____ Organic produce, free-range eggs, and copacetic chickens are just hype.

_____ I give my kids cereal for a healthy snack.

_____ Diabetes runs in my family. If I get it, I get it.

_____ I've heard about stem cells, but I think they're illegal in my state.

Scoring

0–2 items checked: You can still share this book at your next family celebration.

3–5 items checked: You will most certainly find valuable surprises in this book.

6+ items checked: You will want to get sticky notes and a highlighter.

PART I

The Root of All Evil

CHAPTER 1

When Sugar Poisoning Hits Home

—the nerve of it

"Most of my patients are fat, lazy, and confused."

That's the kind of remark I often hear from my other doctor colleagues after we wrap up a successful surgery—say, playing tennis, attending seminars, or sitting in the bar afterward work. Many of the physicians I know are pissed, and I can't say that I blame them.

Because I'm pissed too.

Let's say that my first patient of the day is a plump young woman with Morton's neuroma (an extreme and painful sensitivity on the ball of the foot). Worst case can only be relieved by stripping out the nerves and removing the fibrosis[4]—causing a permanent

---

4   A mass of connective scar tissue caused by trauma. Your body has literally created a stone for you to walk upon.

unnatural splaying of the third and fourth digits. Morton's neuroma, by the way, is frequently attributed to wearing high heels.[5]

I review her medical history as she sits in my office, literally crying from the pain she's in and begging me to make it stop. I've been a podiatric surgeon for three decades, and what I *really want* to say is this:

> "You wear high heels because you think they make your legs look thinner. Fine, that's great! Your choice. Meanwhile, you exercise and then reward yourself with Häagen-Dazs® or strawberry daiquiris. Do you not know—or do you not *want* to know—that your condition is created by both high heels *and* sugary treats? Will you believe me, or is every painful step worth the treat?"

Then I ask myself, Will she even believe me if I challenge her to accept the truth? The initial answer may be no. But I keep trying; and more often than not, the message gets through.

Or let's say I've spent a sleepless night after seeing a patient in clinic who was still confused about the importance of taking sugar out of his diet. A great guy, smart and loving to his family, yet one who still doesn't understand *why*—after months of neglecting his diabetic ulcer (a.k.a., being too busy), after ignoring our treatment plan—*why* our only option now is to cut off his toes and maybe half his foot. He's horrified and defiant. After

---

5   In a 2015 study presented by the Royal College of Surgeons, Edinburgh, Andrew Craig reported that the incidence of Morton's neuroma has increased 115% in recent years with most patients being women between the ages of 40 and 69. I've found that 42% of my Morton's neuroma patients also had either metabolic syndrome or diabetes.

skillfully managing everybody else in his life, he tries negotiating his way out of it.

But I'm in some battlefield movie, and I have to say the truth. "If we don't cut it out, the infection will *kill* you."

WHEN SUGAR POISONING HITS HOME

My own path toward becoming *un*-glued began in 1997 when emergency gallbladder removal forced me to reevaluate my diet and my beliefs about what constituted a healthy lifestyle. I'd always gotten plenty of exercise and followed the recommendations in the USDA food pyramid. No one ever guessed how old I was. My basic diet and exercise patterns were consistently on target, and I felt great—right up to the moment I was doubled over by the agonizing pain of a gallbladder attack. Every nerve in my gut felt as if they were on fire. If you've never experienced this (and I hope you haven't and won't), let me just say that, in the emergency room, gallbladder attacks are often mistaken for heart attacks—and vice versa. Think about that.

I was utterly confused as to how this ailment could have happened. All the surgeon seemed to say was "We got that gallbladder out with no problem. Relax. Forget about it; you're fine." Boy, was he wrong; something was still out of whack with my digestive system. I continued to have many of the symptoms of gallbladder disease: gas, nausea, and abdominal discomfort after meals, as well as chronic diarrhea.

Shortly thereafter, I ran into a friend and family physician in the hospital lunchroom. Still looking for answers, I told him about my surgery.

"Well," he said. "You're not exercising it; after all, the gallbladder is a muscle. You should've eaten more. Keep it working. Look at you; you're too thin."

Mind you, he was obese, and his lunch tray was overflowing. I knew intuitively that he was wrong. Years later I'd conclude that I'd been eating so much sugar and inflaming the vagus nerve going to the gallbladder. As a result, it was not fully contracting, not emptying completely, and gallstones developed. Moreover, 50% of people who have their gallbladder removed go on to develop diabetes.

I began noticing the link to my clinical practice. As we were preparing to remove the toe or a leg of a diabetic patient, I'd review the medical history. Often, the patient had had their gallbladder removed 15 or 20 years prior. That's when I realized I could be such a patient in a couple of decades. At that moment, I decided to step out of my silo of podiatric surgery and begin my own research into the science and chemistry of nutrition.

My journey has become a quest to inform the public of the travesties I've observed regarding how medical treatments have and have not evolved. For instance, I question *why* in the U.S., every year, we perform nearly 150,000 amputations of the lower limb unrelated to trauma—meaning due to vascular disease (primarily due to diabetes, a disease everyone agrees is inextricably linked to diet).

Why am I and my colleagues cutting off so many toes, feet, and legs—when we should instead be teaching our patients how to *avoid* the damage that makes such procedures necessary?

I began searching for the answer by studying the accomplishments of Nobel Prize winners—first in medicine (originally called the Nobel Prize for Physiology), then chemistry, and finally physics.[6]

As most school children have been taught, Alfred Nobel was a scientist, inventor, *and* businessman of the late 19th century, whose greatest financial success came from stabilizing nitroglycerin with diatomaceous earth (sedimentary rock that is fossilized remains of tiny aquatic organisms) to create dynamite.[7] So horrified by the destructive powers he had unleashed unto the world, Nobel bequeathed his fortune to the creation of a foundation to reward those who would create a counterbalance—profound benefits to humanity. Since the first award in 1901, there have been more than 600 awards given to nearly a thousand recipients.

A GREAT LEAP FORWARD

My journey was catapulted forward in 2000 when I attended a lecture given by A. Lee Dellon, MD, professor of neurosurgery at the Johns Hopkins University School of Medicine.

The day I met Dr. Dellon, he said to me, "Why do you podiatrists cut nerves out of the foot to relieve diabetic neuropathy?" It was a keen observation because we're the only surgeons who cut a nerve as a means of fixing something.

---

6   Of course, The Nobel Foundation also awards accomplishments in literature, peace, and economics.

7   Interestingly, nitroglycerin had been used by physicians since the 1700s for the treatment of chest pain. Early on, it was rubbed on the chest. Today we prescribe nitroglycerin pills for angina. What does it do? It dilates blood vessels, easing constriction, specifically in those supplying blood to the heart. It was Nobel, with his out-of-the-box thinking and scientific exploration, who came up with a truly original use for it.

I replied, "Because that's what we're taught."

He said, "Well, come down to Johns Hopkins, and I'll teach you about how inflammation puts pressure on that nerve and how removing the pressure removes the pain."

I had already read his magnificent textbook on the topic, but as a surgeon, I had never seen the actual *compression* itself, not until he showed me. I could comprehend what he wrote—I just couldn't visualize it.

Once at his clinic in Baltimore, we spoke to a patient who described the alternating numbness and sharp, painful tingling that I'd heard described by most of my own patients. Then, I scrubbed in with Dellon and attended one of his surgeries—as he went to work relieving the nerve compression in the patient's foot.

There with 3.5 magnification loops attached to my glasses, I looked into the open incision to the spot Dellon pointed out. Imagine a section of fine, petite-point needlework, with tiny threads crossing over threads—a tendon pressing on the nerve.

He said, "Let's move that tendon off and look again."

And there, just beneath the obvious inflammation, was a tiny dent or impression in the nerve wall. The nerve was being compressed by physical pressure. That's what was causing all the pain and preventing signals from being transmitted to the muscle it served. Seeing it was like opening a door to another world.

The best analogy of that treatment is to imagine kids playing with a garden hose. Your little brother is terrorizing everyone with the hose at full force. You run out of sight and secretly stand on the hose, reducing the flood to a trickle. Then when he looks at the nozzle, you lift your foot to relieve the pressure and a gush of water squirts him in the face. It's a mostly harmless trick and easy to laugh about.

In the not-so-fun world of surgery, though, what I wanted to know about Dr. Dellon's "cure" was what was happening bio-chemically. In a process known as the Maillard reaction, protein plus sugar was causing contraction of the tendon and compres-sion on the nerve. Once the compression was removed by Dellon's instrument, the electric conduction within the nerve began again almost immediately. The fluid within the nerve itself, called the axoplasm, started flowing freely.

DOUBLE DOWN IS NOT JUST FOR POKER

The original discussion of what's known as double-crush phe-nomenon was first published by Drs. Upton and McComas in the *Lancet* in 1973. If, for example, there's a subtle compres-sion of the median nerve at your wrist, there is still flow and you have no symptoms. Then, when a second compression occurs, the "double crush" stops the axoplasmic flow, and your carpal tunnel symptoms begin. The doctors observed that multiple compressions along a single nerve add up to excruci-ating, chronic pain. Relieve the pressure, and the flow comes back to normal.

They also observed that when doing carpal tunnel decompressions, many patients also experienced the relief of neck pain because the brachial plexus (a network of nerves extending from the shoulder to the hand) also benefited from restored axoplasmic flow (movement of subcellular structures).[8]

In addition, Upton and McComas noticed that 16% of those patients with carpal tunnel also had diabetes. And the difference with compression caused by sugar inflammation is that relief can't be manipulated. You must get "*un*-glued" by removing the source—either by stripping out the sticky gunk or by stopping your consumption of sugar. Later, we'll learn how stem cells also can accomplish what we've been doing with a scalpel.

THE CHALLENGE THAT INSPIRED

I was lucky enough to study with Dellon when he was first training surgeons on his compression theory and breakthrough surgical technique for carpal tunnel (involving the median nerve of the wrist), followed by the technique to decompress the ulnar tunnel (involving the nerve at the elbow).

In the 1980s, he published his first papers on triple nerve release (decompression) of the lower extremities, and he loved telling the story of how he got there. After he'd successfully treated a woman for debilitating ulnar tunnel, she asked, "You fixed my arm; why don't you fix my leg?"

He told her, "No, that's a different disease."

---

8   That's exactly what chiropractors and physical therapists do, by the way. They manipulate the muscles with short, sharp thrusts to relieve the tightness within a space, axoplasmic flow is increased, and the pain goes away.

And that's what neurologists thought at the time—her leg pain, diabetic polyneuropathy, was thought of as a separate disease. Yet, her simple logic made perfect sense. So, being the consummate scientist, he went to the lab, banded the legs of both diabetic and nondiabetic rats, and figured out that the same mechanism was at work. He proved that the presence of hyperglycemia (the high blood sugar seen in those with diabetes) meant that those rats were more susceptible to chronic compression of the peripheral nerves in their feet.[9]

One day, after hearing the story again, I asked him, "Compression theory works for neuropathy in nerves of the wrist, the elbow, and the foot. So wouldn't this same technique work with *any* neuropathy throughout the body?"[10]

"Oh, I don't know about that," he said. "It's a different disease."

"But why wouldn't it be the same? To paraphrase Gertrude Stein, 'A nerve is a nerve, is a nerve, is a nerve.'"

He answered with a collegial challenge, "Well, why don't you figure it out?"

So, I took him up on it.

---

9   Dellon took a lot of professional grief for that breakthrough, even from some neurologists with prestigious institutions like the Mayo Clinic. They decried his work, saying, "No! It's dangerous. You don't operate on a diabetic because it's an insidious, ascending disease." The critics were right about that observation but wrong about the biochemical effects that caused the nerve to become compressed by excess sugar.

10 As a young student I'd studied the logic of mathematical equations through tautologies: If *a* is true and *b* is true, all things like *a* and *b* are also true. That's a tautology, and it has to do with redundancy. But if *a* is true and *b* is false, then all things like them can be either true or false, and so another factor is at play.

THE NEXT LEAP FORWARD

I was still making my way through the accomplishments of Nobel laurates when I came upon Otto Heinrich Warburg, sole recipient of the 1931 prize in physiology (medicine) for his "discovery of the nature and mode of action of the respiratory enzyme."

In 1944, Warburg was nominated for a second Nobel for his work with enzymes and the mechanics of fermentation—and throughout his career he garnered 45 additional Nobel nominations by contributing to our knowledge of plant physiology, cell metabolism, and oncology. Subsequently, Warburg concluded that cancer cells grow by replacing "the respiration of oxygen in normal body cells by a fermentation of sugar." In other words, cancer is a metabolic mechanism in which cells feed off sugar, specifically glucose.

The hypothesis, called the Warburg effect, fell out of favor in the early 1950s when researchers unraveled the mysteries of DNA, and focus shifted to the theories of gene mutations and the idea that a relentless drive to replicate were at the root of cancer growth.

For decades, Warburg's observations of sugar as a metabolic catalyst were even omitted from medical textbooks. Recently, however, there has been renewed exploration of the Warburg effect, substantiated by further research indicating that unlike healthy cells, cancer cells lack internal control mechanisms for times when nutrients are scarce. Cancer cells have insatiable appetites—a fact documented through positron emission tomography (PET) scans, which can reveal where in the body cancer cells are gobbling up excess glucose. The Warburg effect has led to other hypotheses, such as those from the esteemed biochemist Lewis Cantley, linking

high insulin levels (caused by a sugar-laden diet) to specific mutations found in breast and colorectal cancers.

Now, I was at a true eureka moment—sugar as the sustenance
or even instigating poison for disease. That simple, profound
concept led me to connect the dots and arrive at the global compression theory, which explains not only the death of healthy
cells in the toes and feet of my diabetic patients but cancer and
all disease as well.

People have commented that they think it's unusual for a podiatrist to have come up with that theory. Yet, it's why my experience
at Dellon's surgery was such a blessing, because before then all I
could see were feet that I was operating on—more than a hundred
thousand times in all. I was like the gastroenterologist who only
sees up the gut. But looking through Dellon's lens, I was able to
see the world from outside my own silo. It was a true spiritual
epiphany. Even at that exact moment I thought, "Oh my God, it's
so obvious! How could I have been so unaware?"

Your family doctor, as good as they are, cannot see that connection
without looking through the appropriate lens.

THE SECOND HIT ALBUM IS ALWAYS THE HARDEST

With the publication of my book *Sugar Crush,* I felt pretty good
about things. I was certain that I'd figured out how my patients got
into the painful shape that brought them to my clinic. Problem
solved. Case closed. Instead, I ran headlong into the next set of
formidable challenges.

The first came because "how shit happens"—medically speaking—is not what we physicians learn in school. Instead, we learn how to *identify and categorize* what's laid out before us. Fancy medical nomenclature explains what is clinically observable—for instance, a pheochromocytoma is simply Latin for "a gray-colored tumor." What we do learn is how to fix the problem, most often defined as stopping pain and restoring some form of previous functionality. In the end, if you can't get restoration, you can at least stop pain.

Moreover, I recognize that not all physicians have the luxury of putting on Dellon's lens and seeing the physical indentation in the nerve as he pulls it away from the trauma. Those in particular who aren't surgeons rarely look inside the body at all. They look at a symptom like diabetic polyneuropathy, and they see it differently. Not wrong, just differently.

Yet, what doctors have been taught to see and what they do to keep their offices open can also be diametrically opposed. Physicians are generally intelligent people, so it's easy for them to deduce: "If I see more cancerous basal cells,[11] more patients, I can keep paying my staff and keep my office open. If I see 50 cancerous basal cell patients a day, I can make enough money to keep it all going. If I learn how to stop healthy basal cells from becoming cancerous by telling patients to stop eating sugar… then I'm out of business."

Likewise, if you go to a doctor for psoriasis, they don't get paid to tell you to stop eating sugar. They get paid to give you a laser

---

11 Basal cells are those at the outermost layer of skin. When treated early, most basal cell cancer is curable.

treatment or prescribe a cream, a lotion, a potion, a gismo, a gadget—that's how the medical system works.

Meanwhile, patients often choose a physician affiliated with a giant medical center or hospital complex with excellent ratings. But these facilities make their money off trauma and end-of-life care, while the rank-and-file physician is likely treating symptoms by—and I hate to say it—passing out prescriptions. Moreover, if a patient comes in with a symptom that's covered in a slick TV ad, it's easier to simply write a prescription and make the symptom go away. "You ask for a statin, and I'll write a prescription for a statin." Patients love you for it, and they send all their friends.

However, when the same patients tell you they would die without their chocolate every night, it's much harder (and more time consuming) to convince them that sugar is, in fact, what's creating their symptoms, not to mention hastening their death. Meanwhile, Congress passes legislation literally written by the pharmaceutical lobbyists and slaps on more reporting procedures, thus codifying the cycle.

So, that brings me full circle—back to my suffering patients and the concerns of my pissed-off colleagues.

1. **The Fat**: The stats are obvious.

For decades, the Centers for Disease Control and Prevention has been charting the alarming rate of obesity in adults and children.

Obesity experts Sarah Hallberg and Osama Hamdy[12] discussed this epidemic in the *New York Times* in 2016:

> Roughly one-third of adult Americans are now obese; two-thirds are overweight; and diabetes afflicts some 29 million. Another 86 million Americans have a condition called pre-diabetes.

We have been duped. Go to the grocery store—read the labels— and see for yourself how hard it is to find anything that isn't filled with sugar (especially high-fructose corn syrup) or genetically modified stuff. Then, somewhere in each store you're likely to find a pharmacy where someone waits in line to fill a prescription for drugs to counteract the artificial food in their basket. So, stores not only peddle government-approved contaminants but also make money selling products to cover symptoms of the resultant poisoning.

2. **The Lazy**: Actually, I have neither the inclination nor the right to be judgmental here—especially since, in my experience, the third factor explains how the vast majority of patients who are "lazy about their health" got that way.

3. **The Confused**: And now we come to the heart of it.

---

12 Before her death in 2022, Sarah Hallberg, DO, MS, was medical director of Virta Health and the director of the Nutrition Coalition. Her coauthor, Osama Hamdy, MD, PhD, is medical director of obesity and inpatient diabetes programs at the Joslin Diabetes Center at Harvard Medical School.
   I am a founding member of the Nutrition Coalition. And by the way, since publication of that article the number of Americans with diabetes has risen to **37.3** million; with estimates of over **100** million having prediabetes (also known as frank diabetes). Obesity clocks in at almost **half** of all Americans. Moreover, 97% of the people who died from COVID had either diabetes or prediabetes.

Why *wouldn't* patients be confused about what to eat? Each new scientific food study contradicts the last. "Eat this; never eat that." "These 10 foods to fight cancer." "Beware: Five foods that will probably kill you." Which expert or agency or pharmaceutical ad should you believe? What cures what—and what else just makes it itch more? With all the conflicting information, it seems as if we're all being overeducated into ignorance. Meanwhile, our tax dollars are funding the FDA and every other government organization charged with protecting us. They are taking our money and killing us with it. We are fighting against ourselves.

THE ALL-TOO-SIMPLE SOLUTION REMAINS A TOUGH SELL

When I tell people that all their aches and pains are coming from the damage caused by sugar, they often react with sarcasm: "What's wrong with you, doctor? Don't you like donuts?"

There was a time when I was a dedicated donut eater. However, in medical school we were never taught the truth about sugar, so I had to learn the truth on my own. Now, when I say don't eat sugar that doesn't mean I don't like it—I simply understand it. Now, I see the damage donuts cause.

CAN YOU SEE WHAT I SEE?

For many years I was the only podiatric surgeon in a vascular surgery group of 150 employees. Cleaning out arteries was and remains a booming business. When I spoke about the harm sugar causes our vascular systems, many of my colleagues rolled their eyes. No one wanted to hear that we didn't need to be scraping plaque out of blood vessels if our patients would simply stop eating sugar.

One reason that people find the simple solution hard to believe is because the mind cannot easily perceive what the eye cannot see. I don't expect other physicians or scientists to readily understand, even the brightest of the bright. They are not surgeons; they can be told the theory, but they don't see it physically occurring. And before recent scientific advancements in magnification, nobody could see these mechanisms at work. Nobody could see how the effects of sugar were building up in the minuscule spaces within and throughout the body.

Of course, there are some medical professionals who simply don't care. In a sense, they're like first responders to an accident scene. Not to disparage first responders, but rather than thinking about prevention, rather than preemptively avoiding disease and pain, they're thinking about mitigating the present trauma, focusing solely on fixing what's gone horribly wrong in the patient's natural defense system. To them, it's like lecturing a drunk driver about alcohol when you're busy pulling him out of a car wreck. Their point of view is "My job is to get to the damage as quickly as I can and clean it up."

Meanwhile, the more reward received by all aspects of the health care system—from the hospital industry, to the physicians, to the pharmaceutical industry (and the medical schools they fund), to the legal and regulatory systems that adjudicate liability— the more accident victims they seek to patch up. And so, when everyone is making money off the "accident," there's no incentive to stop it before it happens. The entire medical conglomerate is being enriched at the demise of the recommended dietary guidelines and practices. And we're all guilty.

The same factors rule the artificial-food industry—less real food, more real money. Fortunately, there are a few heroes and heroines, like the brilliant, investigative science journalist Nina Teicholz, who's been trying to convince us for years that the evidence against saturated fats has been misinterpreted. And much of that misinformation is because everyone is financially invested in ignoring the dietary truth—in continuing to just attend to the accident victims.

Case in point—I had a relevant conversation recently with a nurse practitioner who wanted to put one of my surgical patients on a statin drug to control the accumulation of plaque in her arteries. The nurse practitioner's response is understandable if you listen to all the presentations of the pharmaceutical representatives.

I asked, "Do you really understand why all of that plaque is forming in this individual?"

She answered, "It's cholesterol."

"Yes," I said. "But do you understand the pathomechanics of how that happens?"

Her answer was no.

"Well, it's sugar," I said. "Sugar is an adhesive. And cholesterol responds to the inflammation that sugar—of which she eats vast amounts every day—has caused on the wall (endothelium) of the artery. And if the endothelium weren't inflamed (as Dr. Cooke explained to me), it would not become like Velcro, and cholesterol wouldn't stick to it."

The nurse practitioner looked puzzled. So, I tried saying it another way.

"Think of the insides of your arteries as being a wall in your house. If you throw sand at a wall, it won't stick; it'll slide right down. Physics prevails. But if you first paint the wall with a sticky substance, then throw the sand, it will stick—like glue. Once inside your body, sugar becomes the glue—literally in the form of glucose. And when you *throw anything up against it*—cholesterol, inert particles, toxins, malformed cells of any kind—it will stick and wreak havoc. The patient needs to stop eating sugar. She needs to get *un*-glued."

Like our example of the drunk driver, the solution is so simple: Stop drinking (at least) when you drive. And if you're a first responder, realize that simply picking up the broken glass after the accident isn't enough.

This is a book about how too much sugar has screwed us. Glucose is an adhesive molecule that can gum up and tear down every tissue in our bodies—and we label those effects as different diseases. Even if you personally have done everything you know to "be healthy," modern agriculture, the junk-food creation and distribution industry, and Big Pharma all profit by limiting your healthy food options, suckering you in with less than healthy options. And don't rule out genetics in illness. Those who unknowingly carry certain epigenetic genes and eat sugar can expect to get an "-itis"—whether it's arthritis or gastritis, autism or Alzheimer's.

After I've explained all those details to my patients, some will ask, "How do I get *un*-glued?" Stem cell therapies can stop the pain of nerve damage and temporarily soothe a lifetime of sugar addiction—if you have the money. Hundreds of scientists, esteemed members of Congress, and every patient I've ever treated with stem cells calls them *miraculous*. It's why Big Pharma is still fighting to keep them off the market. Meanwhile, there are simple, objective steps you can take. First among them is to stop eating the poison.

Un-Glued will show you why (throughout this book) and how (specifically in chapter 7).

Bibliography

Brand, Richard A. "Biographical Sketch: Otto Heinrich Warburg, PhD, MD." *Clinical Orthopedics and Related Research* 468, no. 11 (2011): 2831–2832. https://doi.org/10.1007/s11999-010-1533-z.

Creager, Mark A., Kunihiro Matsushita, Shipra Arya, Joshua A. Beckman, Sue Duval, Philip P. Goodney, J. Antonio T. Gutierrez, John A. Kaufman, Karen E. Joynt Maddox, Amy W. Pollak, Aruna D. Pradhan, and Laurie P. Whitsel. "Reducing Nontraumatic Lower-Extremity Amputations by 20% by 2030: Time to Get to Our Feet: A Policy Statement from the American Heart Association." *Circulation* 143, no. 17 (2021): e875–e891. https://doi.org/10.1161/CIR.0000000000000096.

Dellon, Arnold Lee, Susan E. Mackinnon, and W.A. Seiler. "Susceptibility of the Diabetic Nerve to Chronic Compression." *Annals of Plastic Surgery* 20, no. 2 (1988): 117–119. https://doi.org/10.1097/00000637-198802000-00004.

de Sousa, Russell J., Andrew Mente, Adriana Maroleanu, Adrian I. Cozma, Vanessa Ha, Teruko Kishibe, Elizabeth Uleryk, Patrick Budylowski, Holger Schünemann, Joseph Beyene, and Sonia S. Anand. "Intake of Saturated and Trans Unsaturated Fatty Acids and Risk of All-Cause Mortality, Cardiovascular Disease, and Type 2 Diabetes: Systematic Review and Meta-Analysis of Observational Studies." *BMJ* 351 (2015). https://doi.org/10.1136/bmj.h3978.

Encyclopedia Britannica. s.v. "Alfred Nobel." Last updated
    March 29, 2024. https://www.britannica.com/biography/
    Alfred-Nobel.

Hallberg, Sarah and Osama Hamdy. "Before You Spend
    $26,000 on Weight-Loss Surgery, Do This." *New York
    Times,* September 10, 2016. https://www.nytimes.
    com/2016/09/11/opinion/sunday/before-you-spend-
    26000-on-weight-loss-surgery-do-this.html.

Jacoby, Richard P. and Raquel Baldelomar. *Sugar Crush: How to
    Reduce Inflammation, Reverse Nerve Damage, and Reclaim
    Health.* New York: Harper Wave, 2015.

Teicholz, Nina. *The Big Fat Surprise: Why Butter, Meat and Cheese
    Belong in a Healthy Diet.* New York: Simon and Schuster, 2014.

Upton, Adrian R. and Alan J. McComas. "The Double Crush in
    Nerve-Entrapment Syndromes." *The Lancet* 2, no. 7825
    (1973): 359–362. https://doi.org/10.1016/S0140-6736(73)
    93196-6.

CHAPTER 2

Dead Is a Very Bad Symptom

—*what too much glucose does to your body*

Philadelphia, winter, 1967. Hospital of the University of Pennsylvania. A magnificent facility, established in 1751 by Dr. Thomas Bond and Benjamin Franklin "to care for the sick-poor and insane who were wandering the streets of Philadelphia." I was a young student showing up for my first autopsy.

Moving through a long gray hall with overhead fluorescent lights and into a stairwell that echoed as my classmates and I clamored down to the basement, we arrived at the morgue. The room itself was predictable: cold with hard, shiny surfaces—tiled walls, marble slabs, porcelain sinks, and metal drains in the floor for when somebody else would wash away the blood.

What struck me were the bodies. Not at all like the chemically preserved cadavers we'd learned to dissect in anatomy labs, the ones you could steel your mind to and almost make impersonal. Bodies on these slabs were the *newly dead,* recognizably real bodies, naked and exposed.

The pathologist began by sawing open the top of the cranium and lifting out the brain, which she then weighed and prepared for dissection. Quickly and methodically, she made the classic Y-shape incision you've probably seen on TV—from the top of each shoulder, meeting at the sternum and extending down to the pubic bone.

We crowded around as the doctor led us through the procedure. It was her job to uncover the mystery of how and why this person had died. In doing so, she would take the body apart bit by bit to interpret accumulated damage: removing, dissecting, and culturing every microorganism in someone who'd been alive just hours before. She would use these clues to make a final diagnosis.

Late in the procedure, she turned and asked me to describe a small mass on top of a kidney. I was caught off guard.

"Well, it looks like a gray-colored thing," I said. "A mass," I added gathering my thoughts.

She replied. "Not bad. You've just described a pheochromocytoma, Latin for 'a gray-colored tumor.'" She plopped the kidney into a stainless steel dish as if saving it for a closer look later.

From that moment on, I understood how the nomenclature of medicine works: It's the report of an *effect*. It's also mostly in Latin, usually derived from the ancient Greek, so the name of an illness or condition sounds more important. But it's still an observation or literal description.

For example, in the early 1900s, German pathologist Felix Jacob Marchand opened an artery, turned to his colleagues, and said something to the effect of "What's all this hard gunk inside?" He named the hardened gunk "atherosclerosis." *Atheroma* is ancient Greek for "gruel," or "gunk;"[13] and *sclerosis* is medieval Latin for "hardening." That's what he saw—an observation, and a good one. But it's not a diagnosis—the name has nothing to do with the root *cause*.

As a podiatric surgeon, I've treated thousands of patients suffering from an obvious effect (or symptom) of damage or disease— peripheral polyneuropathy (usually from complications of diabetes). Obvious because it's extremely painful. Like searing hot needles, it stings, and it burns. It starts in the autonomic nervous system of your legs, feet, or hands—then moves on to the sensory fibers to finally lodge in the motor fibers. The condition signals every part of your body to first feel and then move. Unchecked, it stops the blood flow and leads to gangrene, the death of surrounding tissue. I could treat the effect—amputate the lower limbs and stop the death. But back then I would always wonder what the cause was. For without that knowledge, I was likely to see the same patient again—and again.

For almost 50 years, I've been fascinated by how we can trace someone's health milestones through the scars left behind in their body (carpal tunnel scars, a missing gallbladder, wayward plaque in the arteries, or myocardial infarction—a.k.a., "the big bang"). We can also trace milestones through clinical observations when a patient sits before us and we wonder, How does this all connect? What's the cause? And hopefully the most important question: How do we prevent it? Because as I'm certain we all would agree, being dead is a very bad first symptom.

---

13 Technically, it's the accumulation of fatty deposits and scar tissue leading to thrombosis (commonly called blood clots).

WHAT IF YOU COULD SEE YOUR OWN AUTOPSY?

The "Do I Even Need This Book?" Quiz was just for fun, but what do the physical consequences of sugar poisoning *actually* look like? Obesity is obvious if you've got a mirror. But what if you could go deeper? What if you could step forward in time and witness your own autopsy? The very word "autopsy" means "to witness or see with your own eyes." How many big white or red puss-filled globs would you see on your own postmortem organs? How many dark, crusty wounds or patches indicating cancerous foreshadowing? What will the doctor determine that caused your death?

The overwhelming majority of us (93%) will die of what's euphemistically called natural causes. When I was young and learned that a relative had died of natural causes, I always assumed that meant they just got old and wore out. When the government and others keeping track speak of statistical natural death among the almost three million Americans who die each year, they specifically mean death by preexisting chronic disease. Something that's been going on in our bodies, known or unknown, medically treated or ignored for some time. And often an autopsy reveals aggressive diseases that may not have been the direct cause of death but still were the source of great pain and/or dysfunction.

Six of the top seven causes of death among Americans fall into the natural-causes category. Heart disease remains the all-time champ, coming in at approximately 20%. Within the margin of error, cancers are in a virtual tie at 19.5%. The statistics drop precipitously after that: death from chronic lower respiratory disease (primarily caused by smoking and other inhaled pollutants) ranks third at 5%, stroke at 4%, while Alzheimer's and diabetes tie for fifth at approximately 3%.[14]

Some of us are afraid of dying and are perhaps even in complete denial that it will happen. Some are young and healthy enough to not even think about it. For the majority—I like to call us the ever optimistic—it's time to take a quick, imaginary tour of the kinds of damage that occur when you've spent a lifetime consuming too much sugar. Where has all that sugar accumulated, layer by layer, year by year? The following three-step reality check will not only be initial motivation to answer the question but will also serve as a benchmark for measuring future success.

Step 1: Look in the Mirror

In an actual autopsy, the pathologist first examines the exterior of your body, and so your imaginary autopsy should begin with a head-to-toe look in the mirror. Your own mirrored reflective investigation—the once-over.

• Are you beginning to look like your grandparents?

____ Yes ____ No

Have you already had some of the "-itises" and "-ectomies" they experienced? Dermatitis, colitis, tendonitis, appendectomy, loose and crepey skin that lacks resilience and tone? Answering yes could mean that such conditions are genetic, or it could mean

---

14 According to the CDC, accidents (unintentional injury) slip in between respiratory disease and stroke.

you're experiencing a familial tendency because your lifestyle is very similar to or exactly the same as that of your grandparents or parents and siblings. Or are your own conditions unique to you? How much do you have no control over, and how much might be of your own making? Researchers in the field of epigenetics are searching for the answers to these questions. I'll discuss this area more thoughtfully in later chapters, but for now, a synopsis gets us started.

EPIGENETICS

Occasionally, when I'm explaining my theory of sugar poisoning, someone says to me, "Hold on, doc. I drink bourbon and eat chocolate all day every day, and I'm as healthy as a horse."

And sometimes it's true. There are some individuals who seem predisposed to longevity. Regardless of the nutritional and environmental assaults they inflict upon their bodies—they, their progenitors, and their offspring survive well into their 90s and 100s.

It's been a long-held belief that genetics are fixed and immutable—to a certain degree. And that qualifier is an important proviso, because the relatively new science of epigenetics now tells us that this basic blueprint—the one we come into life with—is constantly changing. Epigenetics is the study of how behavior and environment affect the ways in which genes *work*—how and why they turn off and on.

Isn't that premise the logic of evolution? And so, while we each may have a propensity for specific diseases such as multiple sclerosis, gallbladder malfunction, or kidney failure, epigenetics alters our traditional perception of disease. It is not immutable and unchangeable. Rather it is dynamic and epigenetic—sometimes occurring rapidly on the evolutionary timeline.

One such example is the genetic mutation ALDH2*2, which affects nearly 560 million people (8% of the world's population) including an estimated 45% of East Asians. People with this variant, also known as the Asian Glow, lack a specific enzyme necessary to metabolize alcohol. Consequently, consuming even a small amount of alcohol can cause such individuals to immediately experience rapid heart rate, headache, and a flush reaction presenting as a bright-red coloration on the face. If consumption continues, to the age-old question of nature or nurture, epigenetics suggests nurture plays a larger role than previously imagined.

Unmetabolized alcohol then builds up in the blood, leading to higher incidences of coronary artery disease, stroke, osteoporosis, and numerous cancers of the digestive system. Forensic scientists believe the variant originated from a single founder in southeastern China—as recently as 2,000–3,000 years ago.

Scientists continue to increase our knowledge of environmental mechanisms that can switch your genes on and off, drastically affecting your health and even passing their new formulations on to your children. We see the effect clearly in the linkage between a pregnant woman's exposure to environmental toxins (especially in her gut microbiome) and the health of her child.

After WWII, researchers in Holland determined that children born of mothers who experienced war-related famine had higher incidences of heart disease and obesity. And let's not be squeamish: War-related famine means eating rats, cats, and grass. More recently, we've learned that adults who were exposed to famine in utero have a significantly higher incidence of schizophrenia. Colorectal cancer was one of the first diseases directly linked to epigenetics.

I have spent my career coming to the conclusion that sugar interacts negatively with gut bacteria, causing inflammation and cellular trauma, leading to neuro destruction within the peripheral organs—toes, brain, gallbladder, pancreas, and so on. The more sugar you eat, the more your gut is triggered to stimulate destructive epigenetic change.

For example, I'm reminded of a 40-year-old patient with severely painful peripheral neuropathy—nerve destruction in the feet and legs. When I asked about her consumption of sugar and processed foods, she told me that everyone in her family got diabetes in their 50s, so she was eating as much sugar as she could before it was too late.

In other words, my patient was exacerbating what *may have been* a genetic or familial pattern. More importantly, stopping her intake of sugar did relieve her neuropathy, and she's yet to develop full-blown diabetes.

YOU ARE WHAT YOU EAT—AND IT SHOWS

What else would the pathologist see as clues to what you've been eating? Or put another way, what developing diseases lurk within? Continue with the self-autopsy evaluation.

- Do you have wrinkles, age spots, yellowed fingernails, nail fungus, skin tags, or gnarled joints?

  ___ Yes ___ No

- Has your optometrist mentioned emerging cataracts?

  ___ Yes ___ No

- And have you dismissed such by telling yourself, "That's just aging?"

  ___ Yes ___ No

Actually, all are the direct result of something called the Maillard reaction, which is one of three complex chemical reactions discussed fully in a later chapter. But for now, it's enough to know that in the human body, Maillard causes glycation—a process in which glucose (sugar) reacts with proteins, fats, or nucleic acids (DNA) to produce advanced glycation end products—aptly nicknamed AGEs.

These damaged, cross-linked proteins become stiff and malformed, producing visible and destructive scarring, both inside and outside your body. In the ever-fascinating cosmic schema, it's the same delicious brown reaction you see when you roast corn on a grill or crisp up turkey skin in a hot oven. Standard phraseology in the pathologist's report: "The patient appears older than their physiologic age." A body that's generally free of sugar or toxins breaking through the gut barrier[15] still will age, just more slowly.

Alive and looking in the mirror, you can do something the pathologist can't easily reconstruct—it's a little test I've seen veteran anesthesiologists use before putting a patient under. Place your hands tightly together in the universal prayer position. Then bring them up to eye level. Do you see light peeking through your palms and extended fingers? If not, you have very minimal Maillard reaction. If your fingers or palms are not touching, and you can see light, you're presenting a symptom of Maillard, contracture of the soft tissue. The anesthesiologist then knows if and to what degree your airway may be constricted and whether intubation will be easy or difficult.

Yellowed fingernails are also a marker for the Maillard reaction. What's at work could be a fungus, or it could be deposits of pentosidine, a chemical reaction occurring when sugar causes proteins to break down. Pentosidine also fluoresces under ultraviolet light.[16]

- Do your finger or toenails have deep horizontal or transverse indentations?

    ____ Yes ____ No

---

15 Of course, the gut is a tube from your mouth to your anus, filled with trillions of individual bacteria (the microbiome) from about 200 different species—some essential and some destructive—each of which, through the process of digestion, delivers nutrients and toxins to every part of your body. Later chapters will consider the toxins—those you ate willingly and others placed in your food unbeknownst to you.

16 The instrument used most often by dermatologists in the detection of fungus and pentosidine is called a Wood's lamp. In my home state of Arizona, we use Wood's lamps to find scorpions, but that's another story.

Beau's ridges were first chronicled in 1846 by French physician Joseph Honore Simon Beau, and they are telltale representation of various diseases, including undiagnosed myocardial infarction, liver disease, malnutrition, severe infection, and other metabolic disruptions (particularly diabetes.) They're also caused by a diverse range of trauma, from smashing your finger in a kitchen drawer to chemotherapy.

Finally, and most importantly, take an honest look at your overall corporeal form—your body.

- Are you lugging around 20, 40, or more extra pounds? Particularly belly fat?

    ___ Yes ___ No

When you're spread out on the autopsy slab, regardless of what you've done or not done to date, excess weight is impossible to ignore. Obesity in this context is not about judgment, fat shaming, living well and with nobility, or any of the other complexities you know too well. However, be it tangential or causative—obesity is the most obvious morbidity factor bringing you to the table.

Step 2. Analyze Your Behavior

- Are you taking prescription medications? How many? Enough to require a pill organizer? And does the drug's warning label cite catastrophic side effects, such as "may cause serious internal bleeding, suicidal thoughts, anal leakage, or sudden death if taken with alcohol"?

    ___ Yes ___ No

Often such medications, although well intended, are merely treating symptoms while masking the real cause of disease.

THE TOP MEDICATION PRESCRIBED IN THE U.S. IS...

The answer can get rather complicated, because as Bill Clinton reminded us, it depends upon what your definition of "is" is. Is it according to numbers of prescriptions sold, or is it measured by dollars spent? Do we prefer apples and eat them more often, or do oranges simply cost more? We can only piece together the evidence to get a general picture. According to The Kaiser Family Foundation, 4.3 trillion prescriptions were filled in the U.S. during 2014. Meanwhile, as reported in the *Wall Street Journal*, the Centers for Medicare and Medicaid Services estimates the cost as having spent $103.7 billion in 2013, with the top 100 drugs equaling 60% of the nearly 3,500 individual drugs prescribed. These and other reports bring us to a consensus top five hit list (without verifiable rank):

- Nexium˙ (for heartburn and gastrointestinal disorders)
- Crestor˙ (for cardiovascular disorders, including lowering cholesterol)
- Humira˙ and Enbrel˙ (for arthritis and other inflammatory diseases like IBD, Crohn's disease, and ulcerative colitis)
- Abilify˙ (an antipsychotic)
- Advair Diskus˙ (for asthma)

Unless you're a pharmacist, how can you sort this out? Just pick a drug and go to the manufacturer's website. For example, at the website www.Nexium.com you will find warnings about this acid reflux medication. "Do not use if you are allergic to esomeprazole."[17] "Do not use if you are taking blood-thinning medicines…antifungal or anti-yeast medicines…heart medicine… anxiety medicines…immune system medicines…medicines for HIV infection…or arthritis medicines." "Stop use and ask a doctor if you get…[among other things]…diarrhea."

And in a profound convolution, some of the medications you take for one disease can lead to different ancillary diseases. Let's look at one set of such drugs: those that are designed to reduce cardiovascular risk but that can also predispose you to develop diabetes.

- Thiazides—the diuretics, which revolutionized the treatment of hypertension, irrefutably increase your risk of type 2 diabetes.
- Beta-blockers—impair the release of insulin.
- Statins—lead to the progression of diabetes.

I am neither antimedication, nor antimedical advancements; but suppose you were able to stop the use of any drug by simply altering your diet? Not only is the proposition possible for most patients, but considering diseases caused by sugar and in concert with other dysfunctions within the gut microbe, opting in is highly recommended.

Let's get back to your self-evaluation.

---

17 And how on earth would you know that? It's the generic name for Nexium, by the way.

- Have you ever misplaced your keys or eyeglasses, blaming it on a distraction; entered a room and not remembered why; or come home from the grocery laden with goodies but lacking the single item you went there to buy?

____ Yes ____ No

While there may be other causes, researchers at the Rush University Medical Center in Chicago determined that cognitive impairment could occur up to 18 years before the clinical diagnosis of Alzheimer's. Those findings are nothing to ignore.

- Do you put sugar in your coffee? Have a frozen pastry in the fridge? Or eat Cocoa Puffs˚ with skim milk for dinner when you're really exhausted?

____ Yes ____ No

- Are you intolerant to gluten, often constipated, or always have loperamide HCl (Imodium˚) at the ready for diarrhea?

____ Yes ____ No

- Do you smoke cigarettes, cigars, or a pipe?

____ Yes ____ No

Check yes twice if you sneak around or still think you're cool.

Enough of the veiled indicators. Let's get on with your imaginary autopsy.

Step 3. Imagine What's Inside

Maybe you got a gold star on your mirrored reflective investigation, and you're perfect on the outside, in your mind at least. You look okay, things are neatly packed inside, but the outside is only the surface. What's going on inside? Things you've never imagined will cause pain or distress.

It's time for the internal exam. You can do this; no reason to be squeamish. Even with the brain revealed and the big Y incision, know that there won't be as much blood as you might fear because you'll have no blood pressure, nothing pumping through your veins. Your heart has stopped. That knowledge certainly helps with viewing, so a pathologist can find tracers of existing chronic disease, long influenced by disorder in your gut microbiome—even if never officially diagnosed. If your death were the result of one of the top six natural causes mentioned earlier, what would you see?

1. Heart Disease

Heart disease is an umbrella term describing many conditions, resulting from lifestyle, infection, and congenital factors. The most common and relevant to our discussion is coronary heart disease in which the interior walls of one or both of your exterior coronary arteries thicken and constrict, most often because of a sticky plaque that accumulates and eventually hardens, causing scar tissue and a blockage or embolism.

Damage of this kind is easily spotted in an autopsy, either by touch or looking at a cross section of the arterial wall. Blockage can also occur from blood clots (caused by medicines, trauma, and genetic mutations), as well as tumor tissue or, rarely, an air bubble. In any case, the free flow of blood is inhibited, and heart muscle tissue, starved of oxygen and nutrients, reacts violently to the assault.

Most of us already have quite a lot of built-up plaque (atherosclerosis), and autopsies of young soldiers in WWII, the Korean War, and Vietnam showed that such buildup regularly begins in your early 20s.

How does all this debris end up in your bloodstream in the first place? Despite what you've been told in recent decades, this major form of heart disease is caused not by cholesterol but rather by the sugar and high-fructose corn syrup in your diet.

I'll go into detail in chapter 7 but, just to repeat the quick version, sugars cause inflammation to the inner lining of your blood vessels, and your body's miraculous attempts at self-healing create the buildup. Sooner or later, the result is a coronary event of major or minor magnitude. In fact, a massive coronary event is quite recognizable during an autopsy, and pathologists have likened the appearance to the multiple irregular lines on a cracked egg. During a genuine autopsy, the pathologist may even stick a finger in the pulmonary artery connecting the heart to the lungs, feeling around for a dislodged blood clot.

I'd like to step out of our imaginary autopsy for a moment to emphasize a word of prevention. Coronary heart disease is progressive, and much like the tremors before a big earthquake, it gives off early-warning signals such as: chest or back pain, numbness or tingling, and shortness of breath. Too many of us ignore or shake off the warnings, continuing to put on weight and put off exercise. The symptoms in women also include seemingly unrelated signals such as: heartburn, malaise, heart flutters, and loss of appetite. Researchers are still trying to figure out exactly why.

2. Cancers

Cancer also is an umbrella term describing more than 200 conditions with thousands of suspected points of origin. But, universally, cancer displays as the uncontrolled division of abnormal cells. In this book, I'll be focusing on those cancers directly related to dietary/environmental factors and the linkages that doctors have established between certain conformational diseases[18] such as type 2 diabetes, Alzheimer's, Parkinson's, and possibly obesity itself.

Normally, you can see—under a microscope, that is—that living cells are active, darting back and forth. Cancer cells (be they smaller or larger than others in the region) are easily identifiable as they frantically invade their healthy neighbors. Like swollen ticks, their central cores (nuclei) grow large and darken because of a glut of DNA.

If death has been the result of any form of cancer, the autopsy—much like a battlefield—would instantly reveal the carnage. The path of destruction is gross and thorough, with random clusters of lumpy tumors of varying sizes. Most are white and almost

---

18 In a conformational disease, protein strands fold back in upon themselves. A pathologist can easily see these telltale cells under a microscope as they're irregular or misshapen and accompanied by tiny lesions.

bursting, some red with inflammation—all surrounded by blackened, dead tissue.

Many health practitioners and family members of cancer patients speak of its distinctive "rotting-flesh" smell. Researchers at the University of Pennsylvania Vet Working Dog Center are training dogs to detect the smell of tissue in the early stages of ovarian cancer (fourth leading cause of cancer death in women). The dogs have successfully identified cancerous tissue in 100% of the trials.

3. Chronic Obstructive Respiratory Disease (COPD)

Chronic obstructive respiratory disease (COPD) is also a collection of diseases, primarily emphysema (in which the delicate air sacs in your lungs are damaged, thus preventing adequate intake of oxygen) and chronic bronchitis (in which the spongy lining of your lungs' airways is red and swollen). The primary cause of COPD is smoking any substance,[19] which puts you at a risk *12 times higher* than if you were walking around breathing just the other air pollutants the rest of us are.

The sad story about COPD is that once the damage has occurred, it cannot be reversed short of a lung transplant.

4. Stroke (Cardiovascular Disease)

A stroke occurs when oxygen and blood reach an impasse or blockage in an artery of the brain, and it involves the same mechanics as those occurring in a heart attack. As in all science, we make the language as complicated as possible—not because we wish to confound the patient but because we wish to be precise.

---

19 In early research regarding the nicotine/cannabis "comparables," nicotine simply had
    the distinct disadvantage of being chemically addictive.

Basic nomenclature includes these terms:

- Ischemic stroke: when arteries to the brain are blocked or clotted.
    - caused by atherosclerosis: the same thickening (a.k.a., scarring) that occurs in coronary heart disease.
- Hemorrhagic stroke: when an artery leaks or ruptures, thus hemorrhaging blood into brain tissue.
    - caused by an aneurysm: a bulging (or ballooning) bursting in a weakened space on a blood vessel (usually intracranial or cerebral artery).
- Ministroke: a transient ischemic stroke in which the blockage is temporary and damage to the brain isn't permanent.

5. Diabetes

In 1981, I was asked by the surgeon general of Taiwan to travel to Taipei. They were alarmed at the increasing incidence of type 2 diabetes in their culture. I met with Luke Chu, an MD, PhD in pharmacology, four-star general in the military, and president of the National Defense Medical School. After many subsequent trips, we've become good friends.

Dr. Chu and other medical officials didn't even have terminology to describe what they were observing—but they knew it was new and horrifying. One night after a presentation, I noticed a TKK Fried Chicken franchise across the street from my hotel, and it reminded me of "the colonel."

On the menu I found fried chicken, roast chicken, sweet potato fries, soft drinks, biscuits, and plenty of desserts. That's when

I connected the dots. Since then, American-style fast food has saturated urban Asia—from Big Macs in Jakarta to Pizza Hut in Singapore to Dodger Dogs in the Welcome to LA Café in Hong Kong. In Taiwan, the rate of diagnosed diabetes has increased exponentially, rising from "barely identified" on my first trip in 1981 to 1.7 million cases within a population of 23.4 million in 2014. As I've said, destruction of the gut biome occurs terrifyingly fast.

However, our first question should be "What is Diabetes?" While there are rare forms of diabetes—chemically or surgically induced, as well as latent autoimmune diabetes—most cases fall into three categories:

- type 1, in which the body's immune system destroys the cells within the pancreas, the organ that makes insulin.
- type 2, in which a person has too little insulin or cannot process insulin.
- gestational, which can occur in pregnancy if a woman's hormones interfere with insulin production.

I'll be concerned in this discussion with what's called type 2 diabetes,[20] the overwhelmingly prevalent form, and the culprits surrounding its causes, progression, and control. Type 2 diabetes is a conformational disease in which damaged protein strands fold back upon themselves. We have much vetted science telling us type 2 diabetes is directly related to diet and sedentary lifestyle. And while you wouldn't be able to "see" it in your imaginary autopsy, for more than a century, pathologists have used microscopic samples from the pancreas to spot a telltale

---

20 I personally believe that what others label as types of diabetes are just dots on the continuum of epigenetics, but I'll discuss my thinking fully in chapter 7.

misshapen protein glob (called an amyloid) that profoundly disrupts the production of insulin.[21]

Diabetes is also the primary contributor to other health crises (sometimes called comorbid conditions) including these:

- heart disease
- cancers of all kinds (specifically pancreatic, prostate, and breast)
- stroke
- kidney disease
- hypertension
- blindness
- neuropathy (the painful destruction of nerves in the extremities) and associated amputations
- Hyperosmolar hyperglycemic nonketotic syndrome (leading to severe dehydration, seizures, and coma)
- gastroparesis (damage to the vagus nerve leading to delayed gastric emptying—meaning your gut stops working, and you die).

In years past, most forms of diabetes occurred slowly and over time. That's why type 2 once was considered a disease of old age. That's all changed. We've now identified a condition clinicians call prediabetes, which is most certainly identifiable as apparent obesity in your imaginary autopsy. (Individual researchers and scientists may call it metabolic syndrome, syndrome x, or impaired glucose tolerance.)

---

21   In the pancreas, these are found in the islets of Langerhans, the clusters of cells producing insulin. Amyloidosis can also be found in other organs, including the brain—where they are a marker for Alzheimer's.

Double-check those early self-evaluation questions. Now consider these:

- Have you recently had a blood test?

  ___ Yes ___ No

- Did you understand any of the scores for triglycerides, blood pressure, HDL and LDL cholesterol, or your fasting blood sugar levels?

  ___ Yes ___ No

Don't worry about the second question. In prediabetes, these quantitative values can be fuzzy. Your physician may gloss over them, sometimes prefacing with something like "Your numbers all look good; no worries." However, that conclusion may not be the whole story—which we're going to explore. For now, here's a quick primer on the markers of metabolic syndrome.

SYMPTOMS OF PREDIABETES

1. Obesity.

2. High triglycerides. These tiny fat droplets play a large role in putting on weight, clogging your arteries, and increasing the inflammation leading to heart attack and stroke. The National Cholesterol Education Program (via a subdivision of the National Institutes of Health) sets the guidelines for triglyceride levels.

Normal level   =   less than 150 milligrams per deciliter (mg/dL)[22]

Borderline   =   150 to 199 mg/dL

High   =   200 to 499 mg/dL

Very high   =   500 mg/dL or more

3. High blood pressure (hypertension) or taking medication to treat it. If your blood pressure is 130/85 or higher, or if you're already taking medication to lower it, you're showing one of the classic symptoms of metabolic syndrome.

4. Low HDL cholesterol. HDL is the so-called good cholesterol because it helps remove the "bad" LDL cholesterol from your blood. Having HDL cholesterol *less* than 50 mg/dL for a woman, or *less* than 40 mg/dL for a man, is a sign of metabolic syndrome.

5. High fasting blood sugar or taking medication to treat high blood sugar. If your fasting blood sugar is consistently high, or if you're already taking medication to bring it down, you have metabolic syndrome.

The American Diabetes Association cites the following fasting blood sugar levels:
 o Normal = less than 100 mg/dL and preferably between 75 and 80 mg/dL
 o Prediabetes = 100–125 mg/dL
 o Diabetes = 126 mg/dL or higher

---

22 Mg/dL is the unit of measurement for mass concentration of a substance in a liquid or gas (in this case blood). It stands for milligrams per deciliter. One tablespoon is approximately 15 milligrams. Approximately 6.76 tablespoons equals one deciliter.

If you have two of these markers, you're now in the same dangerous health situation as about 25% of all American adults—and 40% of American adults over age 50.[23] You are likely to become one of the 29.1 million Americans diagnosed with type 2 diabetes.

Yet, far too often, the numbers can be misleading. A family physician may simply check the numbers, find them to be in "normal range," and declare you to be healthy. However, if they never ask about your diet, you could still be well along the path to developing neuropathy, eye problems, kidney disease, and any other number of painful diseases, including sudden death from heart disease.[24] Your only recourse is to change your behavior now.

DIABETES AND THE DOUBLE WHAMMY

We have decades of research confirming that, for the most part, obesity, sedentary lifestyle, diet, and stress contribute significantly to the progression of metabolic syndrome—onward into type 2 diabetes and the inevitable demise of a perfectly functioning pancreas.

If we were in a poker game, it'd be as if someone with type 1 diabetes had been dealt a poor genetic hand and played it brilliantly; while someone with type 2 had been dealt a brilliant genetic hand and played it poorly, thereby grasping defeat from the jaws of victory.

The number of individuals affected is growing faster than you might imagine. Speaking at the 2015 annual meeting of the

---

23 That number is roughly 86 million.
24 Of patients having a first heart attack, 65% also have metabolic syndrome.

European Association for the Study of Diabetes, Dr. Michael Yafi, director of pediatric endocrinology at the University of Texas, Houston, reported the case of a three-year-old child in his clinic being one of the youngest individuals ever diagnosed with the type 2 form of the disease. Weighing 77 pounds, the girl tested negative for the antibodies seen in type 1 (or childhood diabetes).

Her condition is predictable considering the *junk* we are feeding our children and grandchildren. In the HBO film series *The Weight of the Nation*, we hear a chilling prediction: if we continue on this current cultural path, a child born today will have a lifespan shorter than those of their grandparents.

Dr. Julie Wei, a pediatric ear, nose, and throat specialist at the University of Kansas, refers to the "milk and cookie" disease. After years of treating children with upper respiratory and ear infections who did not respond to standard medications, Dr. Wei concluded she was seeing a syndrome that mimicked actual illness and disease. She concluded it was coming from a diet of "milk and cookies"—all the fruit juice blends put in baby bottles, chocolate milk, and especially sweet treat rewards for good behavior. Parents and grandparents of her patients were dispensing far too many sugary and dairy snacks, particularly at bedtime. She cites symptoms of milk and cookie syndrome as: "chronic stuffy nose, nasal congestion, chronic runny nose, cough, sinus infections, sore throat, recurrent croup, allergies, and asthma."

All of those indications are brightly glaring warning signals of diabetes in training. I believe sugar is attacking the vagus nerve— direct conduit from the gut to the brain, with side trips to the glossopharyngeal nerve in the tongue and pharynx, and to the olfactory nerve located within the nose. Particularly at bedtime, gastroesophageal reflux and laryngopharyngeal reflux can occur, further compromising the gut microbiome. It's as if the child's body is screaming, "STOP already!"

The good news regarding the toddler in Houston with type 2 diabetes was that because of early detection, appropriate therapy, and changes her family made in lifestyle and diet, she lost weight and was off treatment in six months. It's important that we not only change our own diets, but those of our children and grandchildren as well.

If we were to anthropomorphize diabetes, it would be the pernicious little provocateur standing quietly at the edges of a crime scene—watching the first responders and basking in the knowledge that it instigated the microbial bullies, contributing to heart disease and cancer (killers one and two), kicking an organ when it was down, and causing the slow torture and eventual death of the human organism.

It takes effort to manage diabetes and stave off prediabetes. Taking charge of your diet and lifestyle isn't easy. But it's far better than any other option.

6. Alzheimer's Disease.

You probably can imagine what your brain looks like. It's likely you've seen a dramatic presentation or a celebrity chef holding up a pork brain as an example of a delicious source of fatty protein. You know a brain is an intricate globe of ridges and indentations, a lighter shade of gray, and shiny wet.

A more distant metaphor is a large cauliflower. And if you cut a cauliflower in half and open it up, you're in the right mindset. That said, the differences seen in the brain cross sections of a person free from Alzheimer's and one who has experienced the ravages of the disease are immediately apparent.

First, the Alzheimer's brain has shrunk, considerably. The outer layer (cerebral cortex)—charged with thinking, planning, and remembering—is shriveled. Similarly, the hippocampus, an area of the cortex and the place where new memories are formed, is sometimes 10% less than normal capacity. It's why in the end stage of the disease, a person cannot remember how to navigate from the bathroom to the bedroom or from the front yard to the front door. The ridges (gyrus) and furrows (sulcus) on the cortex surface have widened and spread apart—like a flower fully open and in late bloom. Finally, chambers inside the brain mass (ventricles) are noticeably enlarged and filled with more fluid than normal.

Meanwhile, in the healthy brain, orderly proteins called tau line up like railroad tracks at a busy terminal. When the tau proteins are disrupted, they collapse, forming twists and turns. They disintegrate and fall apart as if a bomb had exploded in the depot. Plaque piles on. Nutrients can no longer navigate the cell "tracks," and the cells die. Under the microscope, a cross section of brain tissue will reveal these tangled proteins.

What causes this disruption? That's the key to current research into this horrific disease.

I believe Alzheimer's and a precipitant disease, diabetes, are the result of the global compression in nerves caused by sugar. We know that people with type 2 diabetes are twice as likely as those without it to develop dementia and Alzheimer's. One link, difficult to see in our imaginary autopsy, is the triad between diabetes, Alzheimer's, and degeneration of the olfactory nerves. And yet, a very early symptom of Alzheimer's is a loss in olfactory function—you lose your sense of smell.

Diagnosticians of the past would ask a person if he could detect peanut butter held under his nose. If not, this was a quick, early predictor of Alzheimer's. The olfactory nerve, also known as the first cranial nerve, is directly connected to the gut microbial system—where sugars and other toxins are transmitted. The hippocampus, mentioned earlier, is an integral part of the olfactory nerve nucleus. These two centers are intertwined. First you lose your sense of smell, and then you lose your memory. And unfortunately, the Alzheimer's Association recently revealed research establishing links between neuroinflammation and early onset of Alzheimer's in patients who experienced SARS-CoV-2 and COVID-19 viruses.

MISCELLANEOUS OBSERVATIONS

There are many other diseases easily observable to a pathologist and easily imagined in your virtual autopsy.

- Cancerous and precancerous colon polyps (tubular adenoma)
- IBD, Crohn's disease, and ulcerative colitis
- Gallbladder disease
- Carpal tunnel syndrome and tarsal tunnel syndrome
- Fatty liver disease
- Fibroids and cancers of the breast and prostate

While those conditions may not have been the direct cause of your death, they undoubtedly caused you a great deal of pain and discomfort. All are directly related to sugar poisoning.

A BRIEF WORD ON AGING

I have patients who say to me, "It sucks getting old."

And I often answer, "Well, it shouldn't."

Or a patient might bemoan that she's suffering *because* she's getting old. My answer is that aging shouldn't be about suffering.

Death comes to us all. Except for *Turritopsis dohrnii,* the immortal jellyfish that reproduces itself, every organism has a finite, genetic lifespan. Scientists conclude that for humans, it could be about 120 years. In the meantime, many of us die from chaos, accidental or otherwise. However, most of us don't make 120 years because of *abuse, disuse,* and *disease.*

The point is to be as healthy as you can for as long as you can. And that requires maintenance. When you buy a car, what's the warranty? How long should your car last? Did you follow the rules of basic maintenance? Change the oil, keep it out of the sun, use appropriate fuel, and wash the salt from the undercarriage in wintertime. If not, what do you expect?

Meanwhile, I don't want to keep you up awake all night with dark thoughts of your browning, then decaying, innards. Let's move on to chapter 3 and learn more about the global compression theory and specific disease manifestations.

Bibliography

American Heart Association. Accessed April 16, 2024. www. heart.org.

Bortz, Walter M. *We Live Too Short and Die Too Young: How to Achieve and Enjoy Your Natural 100-Year-Plus Life Span.* New York: Bantam Books, 1991.

Brooks, Megan. "100 Best-Selling, Most Prescribed Branded Drugs Through June." Medscape. August 12, 2013. www. medscape.com/viewarticle/849457www.medscape.com/ viewarticle/849457.

Burch, Martin, and Stuart A. Thompson. "Top Prescription Drugs in Medicare Part D." *Wall Street Journal*, April 30, 2015. https://graphics.wsj.com/medicare-prescription-drugs/.

Charnow, Jody A. "Prostate Cancer Death Risk Higher in Diabetes." Renal and Urology News. January 7, 2014. https://www.renalandurologynews.com/news/urology/ prostate-cancer/prostate-cancer-death-risk-higher-in- diabetics.

"COVID-19 May Damage the Brain in Older Adults." Alzheimer's Association. 2021. https://www.alz.org/news/ 2021/covid-19-may-damage-the-brain-in-older-adults.

"Diagnosis." American Diabetes Association. Accessed April 16, 2024. https://diabetes.org/about-diabetes/diagnosis.

Frühbeck, Gema. "Death of the Teaching Autopsy: Advances in Technology Have Not Reduced the Value of the Autopsy." *BMJ* 328, no. 7432 (2004): 165–166. https://doi.org/ 10.1136/bmj.328.7432.165-b.

Hardy, Kate. "Drug-Induced Diabetes." Diabetes.co.uk. April 24, 2024. https://www.diabetes.co.uk/drug-induced-diabetes.html.

Hayden, Melvin R. "Islet Amyloid, Metabolic Syndrome, and the Natural Progressive History of Type 2 Diabetes Mellitus." *Journal of the Pancreas* 3, no. 5 (2002): 126–138. https://pubmed.ncbi.nlm.nih.gov/12221327.

Heijmans, Bastiaan T., Elmar W. Tobi, Aryeh D. Stein, and L. H. Lumey. "Persistent Epigenetic Differences Associated with Prenatal Exposure to Famine in Humans." *Proceedings of the National Academy of Sciences USA* 105, no. 44 (2008): 17046–17049. https://doi.org/10.1073/pnas.0806560105.

Hirschler, Ben. "Toddler with Type 2 Diabetes Highlights Global Obesity Epidemic." Reuters. September 16, 2015. https://www.reuters.com/article/idUSKCN0RG2YE.

Huxley, Rachel, Alireza Ansary-Moghaddam, Amy Berrington de González, Federica Barzi, and Mark Woodward. "Type-II Diabetes and Pancreatic Cancer: A Meta-Analysis of 36 Studies." *British Journal of Cancer* 92, no. 11 (2005): 2076–2083. https://doi.org/10.1038/sj.bjc.6602619.

International Diabetes Federation. Accessed April 16, 2024. www.idf.org.

Kim, Meeri. "Asian Glow from Alcohol Isn't Just a Discomfort. It's a Severe Warning." *Washington Post*, August 15, 2023. https://www.washingtonpost.com/wellness/2023/08/15/asian-glow-alcohol-gene-mutation-cancer-risk.

Konstantinov, Igor E., Nicolai Mejevoi, and Nikolai M. Anichkov. "Nikolai N. Anichkov and His Theory of Atherosclerosis." *Texas Heart Institute Journal* 33, no. 4 (2006): 417–423. https://www.ncbi.nlm.nih.gov/pmc/articles/PMC1764970.

Kumar, Rajan B., Robert S. Wilson, Jennifer Weuve, Lisa L. Barnes, and Denis A. Evans. "Cognitive Impairment 18 Years Before Clinical Diagnosis of Alzheimer Disease Dementia." *Neurology* 85, no. 10 (2015): 898–904. https://doi.org/10.1212/WNL.0000000000001774.

"Leading Causes of Death." Centers for Disease Control and Prevention. Last updated January 17, 2024. http://www.cdc.gov/nchs/fastats/leading-causes-of-death.htm.

National Heart, Lung, and Blood Institute. Accessed April 17, 2024. www.nhlbi.nih.gov.

Ohara, Tomoyuki, Yasufumi Doi, Toshiharu Ninomiya, Yoichiro Hirakawa, Jun Hata, Toru Iwaki, Shigenobu Kanba, and Yutaka Kiyohara. "Glucose Tolerance Status and Risk of Dementia in the Community: The Hisayama Study." *Neurology* 77, no. 12 (2011): 1126–1134. https://doi.org/10.1212/WNL.0b013e31822f0435.

Osterloff, Emily. "Immortal Jellyfish: The Secret to Cheating Death." Natural History Museum. Accessed April 16, 2024. https://www.nhm.ac.uk/discover/immortal-jellyfish-secret-to-cheating-death.html.

Painter, Rebecca C., Tessa J. Roseboom, and Otto P. Bleker. "Prenatal Exposure to the Dutch Famine and Disease in Later Life: An Overview." *Reproductive Technology* 20, no. 3 (2005): 345–352. https://doi.org/10.1016/j.reprotox.2005.04.005.

"Penn Vet Working Dog Center, Penn Physics, Penn Medicine, and Monell Chemical Senses Center Receive $80K Grant to Fund Study of Ovarian Cancer Detection by its Odorant Signature Using Dogs and E-Sensors." May 1, 2013. PennVet: University of Pennsylvania. https://www.vet.upenn.edu/research/academic-departments/biomedical-sciences/news-events/biomedsci-news/

penn-vet-working-dog-center-penn-physics-penn-medicine-and-monell-chemical-senses-center-receive-80k-grant-to-fund-study-of-ovarian-cancer-detection-by-its-odorant-signature-using-dogs-and-e-sensors.

Pinto, Jayant M., Kristen E. Wroblewski, David W. Kern, L. Philip Schumm, and Martha K. McClintock. "Olfactory Dysfunction Predicts 5-Year Mortality in Older Adults." *PLOS-One* 9, no.10 (2014): e107541, https://doi.org/10.1371/journal.pone.0107541.

Poznyak, Anastasia, Andrey V. Grechko, Paolo Poggio, Veronika A. Myasoedova, Valentina Alfieri, and Alexander N. Orekhov. "The Diabetes Mellitus–Atherosclerosis Connection: The Role of Lipid and Glucose Metabolism and Chronic Inflammation." *International Journal of Molecular Science* 21, no. 5 (2020): 1835. https://doi.org/10.3390/ijms21051835.

"Total Number of Retail Prescription Drugs Filled at Pharmacies." The Henry J. Kaiser Family Foundation. Accessed April 16, 2024. www.kff.org/other/state-indicator/total-retail-rx-drugs/www.kff.org/other/state-indicator/total-retail-rx-drugs.

Wallace, Charles P. "Fast Food in Asia on Fast Track." *Los Angeles Times*, February 9, 1994. https://www.latimes.com/archives/la-xpm-1994-02-09-mn-20882-story.html.

Wei, Julie. "Milk and Cookie Disease." Dr. Julie Wei. Accessed April 16, 2024. https://www.drjuliewei.com/pages/what-is-mcd.

Weight of the Nation. Season 1, episode 3, "Children in Crisis." Aired May 15, 2012, on HBO. https://www.hbo.com/the-weight-of-the-nation/season-1/3-children-in-crisis.

CHAPTER 3

The Dose Is the Poison

—how global compression progresses and conforms

Whether white or brown—organic or packed with pesticides—**sucrose** is the chemical name for refined (table) sugar.[25] Although sugar-filled crops were cultivated in places like the swamps of New Guinea around 8,000 BCE, what we recognize as refined sugar was first recorded about 2,500 years ago in India. From there, it moved to China, to Persia, and to the Islamic nations where it was stumbled upon by European crusaders. It consists of two carbohydrate molecules—our old friend, **glucose**, and a fresh face in our saga, **fructose** (found chiefly in fruits and some vegetables, predominantly beets, corn, and potatoes).

In the 16th century, Swiss physician, chemist, and philosopher Paracelsus coined the phrase "the dose is the poison." And his words are particularly true of sugar.

---

25 Sucrose is also the primary ingredient in fruit juice, milk, honey, molasses, and maple syrup.

Defined by many scientists as a chemical toxin, sucrose is the most damaging ingredient that you routinely welcome into your personal gut microbiome. Once there, it passes unscathed through your gut wall—first causing inflammation of delicate nerve cells—then traversing throughout your body destroying organs, joints, and tissue as it goes. It is ravenously devoured by not only the bacteria and viruses already in your body but cancer cells as well.

Sucrose is blatantly culpable for a host of related neurodegenerative conditions, from diabetes, heart disease, ALS, high blood pressure, multiple sclerosis, obesity, cancer, Alzheimer's, autism, acne, carpal tunnel, psoriatic arthritis, wrinkles, and migraines, as well as devastation of any peripheral organ in the body, including the gallbladder, liver, lungs, spleen, brain…

You get the picture.

Some cultures and peoples don't particularly like sugar. It's pulled out from the back of the cupboard only for celebratory functions or to fill the hummingbird feeders. There's strong evidence that our primordial ancestors rarely stumbled upon wild honey or sugary plants. And apparently some animals, namely cats, can't even taste it.[26] Yet, by all accounts, we Americans love—I mean *really* love—our sugar. It could be said that we wallow in it.

Since 1970, the U.S. Department of Agriculture has been tracking the total annual per-person consumption of sucrose (in the form of cane sugar, beet sugar, corn sweeteners, edible syrups, and honey).

---

26 In a later chapter I'll discuss new research identifying possible genetic links to the flavor itself.

Are you sitting down?

- In 1999, consumption peaked at 153.6 pounds of sugar per person per year.
- The projection for 2023 is 125.8 pounds per person per year.

True, it is a decrease, which shows that some people have been awakened to sugar's harm, but the word about it is spreading at a dangerous snail's pace. Look at it this way: There are approximately 201 teaspoons to a pound of granulated sugar. So, that's 25,286 teaspoons of sugar a year OR a pinch more than **69 teaspoons of sugar a day**!

What's that? You can't believe it? Not you?

HIDING IN PLAIN SIGHT

You may proudly declare that you *never* eat candy, donuts, or derby pie. In fact, you can march away from the office birthday cake in a New York minute. But don't be so smug because high amounts of *secret sugar* can be found *anywhere*. (I was shocked to find a local restaurant that even puts it in the guacamole.) A study at the University of California San Francisco concluded that an estimated 74% of packaged foods contain added sugar—even those also advertised as "healthy" or "natural."

Two flashing neon signs that an ingredient is really a secret sugar:

1. It ends in "-ose."
2. It includes the words "sugar," "syrup," "juice," "nectar," or "concentrate."

When checking lists of ingredients, you may see names such as these:

- Agave nectar
- Barley malt
- Brown sugar
- Rice syrup, malt syrup, date syrup
- Cane
- Corn sweetener
- Corn syrup or corn syrup solids
- Dextrose
- Fruit juice concentrate
- Fructose
- Galactose
- Glucose or glucose solids
- High-fructose corn syrup
- Levulose
- Maltose
- Maltodextrin
- Molasses
- Sucanat
- Sucralose
- Sucrose
- Treacle
- Turbinado

You can also estimate the number of teaspoons of added sugar in a processed food product by dividing the number of carbohydrates by four. We could fill the chapter with charts listing the sugar content of fast-food favorites, but here's an example to illustrate the point: One McDonald's regular cheeseburger contains 33 grams of carbohydrates. That's 8.25 teaspoons of sugar. I'm guessing most is in the bun as I've had patients tell me that after cutting back drastically on sugar, McDonald's hamburger buns taste like donuts.[27]

Meanwhile, the American Heart Association recommends that men consume no more than nine teaspoons of added sugar per

---

27 In 2014, the fast-food chain even experimented with infusing bubblegum flavor into broccoli to make Happy Meals "healthier." It didn't fly with the kids.

day. For women, the number is lower: six teaspoons per day. To sync up with the USDA, these are the recommendations:

- Nine tsp. of added sugar per day (3,285 tsp. or 16.3 lb. a year) for men.
- Six tsp. of added sugar per day (2,190 tsp. or 10.89 lb. a year) for women.

And note this important point: The American Heart Association is saying that six to nine teaspoons of sugar are *over and above* those sugars/carbohydrates found naturally in unprocessed, fructose-packed fruits and vegetables.

DO WE EVEN *NEED* SUGAR AT ALL?

Well, yes, it turns out that we do. Recent technological advancements now allow scientists to probe at a microlevel (50 microns) and study the mammalian glycocalyx, a gel-like, diaphanous network connecting each cell. As the name implies, it's heavily glycosylated (meaning mainly made of sugar). Leonhard Möckl of the Max Planck Institute describes it most simply: "All cells in the human body are covered by a dense layer of sugars and the proteins and lipids to which they are attached, collectively termed the glycocalyx…sweet husks."

The primary purpose of this biofilm is for protection. Otherwise, pathogens like bacteria would easily invade. So, it repels what is harmful to the cell—it's a guardian, a microscopic suit of armor. It also helps in the transmission of intercellular information.

For all this function to happen, you need only to ingest but one teaspoon of sugar at any given time. Any more, and you're starting to gum up the works. Physiology kicks in, triggering the insulin response[28] to clear glucose from the bloodstream. Continue eating more sugar over time, and you're on the slippery slope as your metabolism—overwhelmed by the volume—tries and fails, then tries and fails again to regulate. Your body fights back with inflammation, and physical catastrophes follow. All the while, sugar feeds bacteria, viruses, and cancers and swaddles you in stored fat. Remember Paracelsus—the dose is the poison.

In later chapters you'll learn how stem cells can help you become *un*-glued. However, to *stay un*-glued, and using the American Heart Association guidelines as comparison, I believe you should consume, not 69, not nine, not six—but **one teaspoon of added sugar per day** (or approximately 365 tsp. or 1.8 lb. per year), keeping in mind all sources of sugar.

You don't need to have an interest in the chemistry of it. Just use your good common sense. Begin by purposefully and thoughtfully removing as much sugar from your diet as you can. Commit to it and see if you notice feeling better, moving better, being free of chronic aches and pains. I guarantee that you will. I've already committed my professional life to bringing you this message.

---

28 This insulin response leads to the A1C blood sugar count you've heard about in all the TV commercials for diabetes medication. According to the Centers of Disease Control and Prevention (CDC), a normal A1C level is below 5.7%, a level of 5.7% to 6.4% indicates prediabetes, and a level of 6.5% or more indicates diabetes. Within the 5.7% to 6.4% prediabetes range, the higher your A1C, the greater your risk is for developing type 2 diabetes.

A DEEPER DIVE INTO THE GLOBAL COMPRESSION THEORY

Chapter 1 introduced my global compression theory, which was built upon the nerve-compression theory established by Dr. A. Lee Dellon (1984) that grew out of the work of Upton and McComas (1973).

The Global Compression Theory
Sugar (glucose) = Chronic Inflammation +
Trauma (compression or injury)
= Nerve Damage, Pain, and Dysfunction

The biochemistry of *how* this result happens involves three complex mechanisms, which were fully discussed in *Sugar Crush* and summarized here:

1. The Maillard reaction—a chemical interaction (glycation) that occurs when glucose reacts with proteins, fats, or nucleic acids (DNA), causing scars called advanced glycation end products (aptly abbreviated AGEs). As your immune cells work to break the scars apart, they secrete inflammatory chemicals in a process identical to what happens to turkey skin in a hot oven. On *your* skin, the result is wrinkles and age spots. Imagine what it does to your vital organs.

2. The polyol pathway[29]—a series of chemical reactions by which your body metabolizes excess sugar (either glucose

---

29 It's called a pathway because it is a step-by-step, interconnected progression, in which each step must be triggered by an enzyme (usually a protein).

or fructose) into sorbitol. This related sugar is commercially derived from stone fruits, seaweed, and corn—then repurposed as an "organic sweetener" in countless processed foods, including dietetic candy and imitation crab. Like all sugars, sorbitol draws in water, causing it to swell. Stuck in place, it reduces blood flow to the nerve, starving it of nutrients and oxygen. And if that spot already has tight tunnel nerve swelling, the compression causes the burning pain and numbness of neuropathy.

3. The nitric oxide pathway—a series of chemical reactions beginning in the lining of blood vessels called the endothelium. Here the amino acid (L-arginine) converts to nitric oxide—and this gas relaxes blood vessels, allowing for the free flow of blood.[30]

In *Sugar Crush,* I was the first to theorize how a second amino acid, asymmetric dimethylarginine (ADMA), could cause the same compression in blood vessels that it does in nerves:

An amino acid found naturally in your body ADMA is structurally very similar to L-arginine. We could call them cousins. And so, both ADMA and L-arginine can attach to the enzyme nitric oxide synthase.

When L-arginine attaches, it converts to nitric oxide, and your vessels function the way they should. When ADMA attaches, however, it converts to peroxynitrite,[31] which clogs the conversion and blocks the production of nitric

---

30 So, it's no surprise that nitric oxide and L-arginine supplements have become so popular.
31 The chemical symbol for peroxynitrite is, rather appropriately, OONO.

oxide. (Not good.) Technically speaking, ADMA inhibits nitric oxide synthesis. Too much ADMA in your blood (also linked to insulin resistance) causes your blood vessels to constrict rather than dilate.

...Which reduces blood flow to the nerve—and reduced blood flow means that the tiny blood vessels bringing nutrients and oxygen to your nerves constrict and then clog up.

When I first predicted this 17 years ago, the effect of ADMA had not been confirmed. Now it has by several researchers including the following:

- Achim Burger, MD, and others from the University of Vienna who found that "patients with ICM [ischemic cardiomyopathy][32] or DCM [dilated cardiomyopathy][33] have elevated plasma levels of ADMA compared to control patients."
- Scientists with the Department of Endocrinology, Hebei General Hospital, Hebei, China, who concluded, "Elevated ADMA levels correlate with diabetic microangiopathies such as DR [diabetic retinopathy] and diabetic nephropathy. ADMA may play an important role in the pathobiology of microvascular complications of diabetes."

I connected the dots linking ADMA to Dellon's nerve-compression theory, and my quest illustrates the collaborative and even serendipitous nature of science. As I mentioned in chapter 1, I'd gone to Johns Hopkins to study with Lee Dellon in 2000. Then in 2004,

---

32 Decreased ability of the heart to pump blood.
33 A heart muscle disease causing the left ventricle heart chamber to enlarge, causing the walls to become thin and stretched.

quite by chance, I read an article published by John P. Cooke, MD, PhD, one of the world's leading cardiologists/vascular biologists, who was then a professor of cardiovascular medicine at Stanford. The title of his article asked if ADMA could be an "uber marker" regarding endothelial function. It set off a light bulb!

I texted him: "Dr. Cooke, I think your theory may have something to do with Lee Dellon's compression theory." He called me back in two hours. What busy person calls back a stranger in two hours? But he did. In that conversation, he invited me to come up to Stanford to look at his work, and I took him up on his offer.

Cooke's discovery was that we could measure ADMA (your body's inflammatory marker), and we now have devices to bring more nitric oxide to the system to power a cell's mitochondria to produce more adenosine triphosphate (ATP), which is the actual fuel for the body, providing energy for several metabolic processes and the making of RNA.

ADMA is the inflammatory agent that blocks the autonomic nervous system, causing a cascade of related diseases, including ALS (amyotrophic lateral sclerosis, a progressive neurodegenerative disease that affects nerve cells in the brain and spinal cord). Stem cells can temporarily correct that condition. But if you don't stop eating sugar, the process starts all over again. And by the way, upon hospital admission, high ADMA levels are used to predict the severity and morbidity rates of COVID cases—because it also cuts off the supply of oxygen.

Dellon had his eureka moment in the early 1980s. In 1998, three American pharmacologists, Robert Furchgott, Louis Ignarro, and Ferid Marud, won the Nobel Prize in Medicine for their discovery that nitric oxide is a critical signaling molecule to relax and expand blood vessels. Cooke, the world-famous cardiologist from Stanford, and I were studying the metabolic features of sugar in the early 2000s. And voilà!—sugar plus a protein equals a reaction.

SUGAR AND MULTIPLE SCLEROSIS

"*You Fat-Shaming Bastard* ☺" That's how the email began.

I'd been on a syndicated talk-radio show, *The Higherside Chats*, and at the end of the broadcast, host Greg Carlwood chided listeners who'd become so obese they had to order his promotional T-Shirt in sizes 3X–4X. Several weeks later, he forwarded this email from Keith, one of his listeners.

> Got to tell you I was a little pissed at you and then realized that it was me I should be angry at. I'm one of those people that buys 3X shirts…[and I] was diagnosed with multiple sclerosis…. That day after listening to Dr. Jacoby, I said f-sugar, started a keto diet, and ordered his book. It's amazing how much better I feel now. Feel free to forward this [to him] if you think he'd like to hear the feedback.

One thing was certain: I absolutely wanted to hear more of Keith's feedback. I learned he was then 46 years old, 6'1 in height, and had reached a top weight of 370 pounds. He'd been working in the medical field since 1992, first as a radiologic technologist—working on x-rays, MRI, ultrasound, CT-scans, and then with PACS[34] and digital radiology. From there, he moved into the administration of medical computer systems for hospitals. We began corresponding, and when I asked him about his diagnosis for MS, he had much, much more to say:

> I was driving to another city for a business meeting when, in the boredom of the highway, I guess, I noticed that all my toes felt like they were asleep. I tried wiggling them, moving my free leg as much as I could, and shifting in the car seat; but the sensation wouldn't go away. I pulled into a rest stop and walked around the car. Nothing worked— my toes wouldn't "wake up." I didn't know what was happening, and it scared the hell out of me. I tried putting it out of my mind, but throughout my meeting and the return trip, I could still feel this constant tingling.
>
> The first doctor I went to was completely useless. She gave me a prescription for Lortab, which is a narcotic, and Flexeril, which is a muscle relaxant. Now, I knew better because neither one of these had anything to do with my symptoms. Then I went to a primary care physician who sent me to an orthopedist who was more concerned about a secondary pain in my elbow than he was about why a sharp tingling pain had progressed all over my feet.
>
> He did an ultrasound of my elbow and gave me an injection in my ulnar nerve. That got better, but the treatment didn't fix my neuropathy. The next step was an MRI, and it revealed I had a lesion in the cervical section of my spinal cord, right in my neck. That meant I needed to see

---

34 Picture Archival and Communications System, a medical imaging technology.

a neurologist, leading to other MRIs and two spinal taps (the second because of a hospital error) and the eventual diagnosis of multiple sclerosis. And hell, I was not expecting that. Partially because MS seems to happen more to thin White women. Not fat White men.

Two and a half years later I was taking 800 mg of Neurontin[35] three times a day, along with Voltaren[36] every day. And of course, once a week I take a shot of Anavex.[37] I wasn't happy with taking all these powerful drugs because a) being on Neurontin and b) being on that damn much Neurontin. I decided, "Well, I've got to stop this."

I talked to my doctor, and he said, "Look, none of these first two meds are helping your MS—all they're doing is controlling your pain levels." So, I'd decided to research natural pain treatments. It went well enough that I eventually weaned myself off both the Neurontin and Voltaren.

After my diagnosis, I'd just started eating crap. I was still taking my vitamins…but still, I was eating all the wrong food.

Then I heard you on a radio talk show. The more you talked, the more it resonated, and I started thinking about how much sugar I was eating. You even mentioned MS, and it made sense—if sugar could inflame one nerve, it could inflame all nerves. It all suddenly came into focus;

35 An anticonvulsant medication. Called gabbies on the street, Neurontin (gabaprentin) can produce a euphoric-high like marijuana, along with various harmful side effects.
36 An NSAID, anti-inflammatory painkiller.
37 An interferon commonly prescribed for MS, this drug (self-administered by intramuscular injection) limits the immune system from attacking and destroying the protective coating of nerves.

it was the sugar I was eating. That's what really makes me mad. I'd been seeing a neurologist regularly for almost three years and never once have we discussed diet. The good news is that within two weeks of being off sugar, I felt a 50%–60% decrease in my symptoms.

A few years earlier, I attended a conference on MS, and there I was introduced to Paolo Zamboni, a professor of medicine at the University of Ferrara in Italy. Zamboni became intrigued with MS in 1995, when his wife was diagnosed with the disease. He hypothesized that rather than being an autoimmune disease, MS is actually a vascular disease—that a compromised flow of blood in the veins draining the central nervous system plays a role in its development. He termed this phenomenon chronic cerebrospinal venous insufficiency. He devised a procedure that widens the passage in the jugular vein using a small balloon (angioplasty). To his utter joy, the procedure alleviated his wife's symptoms. That made me think about what might be happening. The vagus nerve lies right on top of the jugular vein. When Zamboni widened (dilated) the vein, the symptoms subsided.

We know that ADMA makes the lining of blood vessels (the endothelium) sticky, causing them to constrict and thus restrict blood flow to the adjacent nerves. This fact led to my own hypothesis that in MS (because of this ADMA-sugar linkage), the vagus nerve becomes stuck to the jugular vein. Inflating the vein and expanding the tunnel could also unstick the vagus nerve, thus stopping the symptoms. Quite notably, the recurrence rate is high with the Zamboni procedure. Recurrence of the constriction could actually reinforce the idea that a diet high in sugar and the resulting sticky ADMA is the real problem.

CONFORMATIONAL DISEASES LIKE MS

MS, like diabetes, Alzheimer's, Parkinson's disease, and arthritis are conformational diseases, a term given to more than 40 diseases that are caused by the accumulation of unfolded or misfolded proteins.

I used to compare the process to what happens with a brand-new travel map. Once it's opened, it can never be refolded correctly to fit neatly back in the glove box (pancreas); but after all the blank stares from my young medical students, I realized the now ubiquitous GPS meant that few had ever seen a travel map.[38]

Now, I describe the concept by talking about socks. I live by myself, so I'm the one who not only wears the socks, but I wash the socks as well. How come I have so many for which I cannot find the mates? Where do they go? Does the washer eat them? Do they run away at night? Still, I keep them, and they get misfolded; they become out of place.

One lone or misfolded sock doesn't ruin anybody's life. But if you can't find the mates to any of them, you've got a big problem. It doesn't happen at a single point in time. It's a continuous, insidious process, and eventually, you have a drawer full of rumpled leftovers only good for dusting the window blinds. We could call it a conformational disease of socks.

Something similar happens at the cellular level. Sugar causes proteins to misfold, creating gaps (lesions), and over time (depending upon the amount of sugar and your genetic makeup), teams break apart, lesions increase, and eventually these "jumbled misfoldings"

---

38 My older patients still get it.

of proteins overwhelm the system. Eventually you will have diabetes, or MS, or any of the other diseases so labeled.

MS has also been categorized as an autoimmune disease—meaning the body's immune system goes rogue, turning against itself to attack various tissues throughout the body. What an absurd concept—the truth is that there is no "autoimmune disease."

Like ripples in a pond, all the markers of chronic inflammation (including fatigue, muscle aches, joint pain, headaches, gastrointestinal complaints, depression, anxiety, and brain fog) are present in patients diagnosed with MS, and all reflect global compression. I believe physicians see an *effect* and think it's the *cause*. The cause is sugar.

The body would not attack itself—that's against design. It's attacking an invader. Take away the sugar, and the attack halts. Instead of recognizing that simple on/off switch, current medical practice is to treat the symptoms, most notably physical pain. Remember Keith's experience.

LET US NOT FORGET FRUCTOSE

It seems the question always comes back to glucose, but as you will recall, refined sugar consists of two compounds. Glucose causes the "gluing"; however, it's **fructose** (especially its evil twin, high-fructose corn syrup or HFCS) that provides a direct causative line to obesity and another condition you'd see in your imaginary self-autopsy: fatty liver disease.

This collection of triglycerides and other thick yellow fats visible throughout otherwise healthy liver tissue leads to fatigue, loss of appetite, weight loss, weakness, fluid retention, bleeding, and shortened lifespan. And a study out of UCLA found that a high-fructose diet even hampers recovery from traumatic brain injury.[39]

HFCS—the American poison we've exported to the rest of the world in everything from Coca-Cola to Dominos—is a deadly liquid form of sugar that makes any food tolerable. Yet as the classic argument goes, fructose and HFCS are processed by the liver—they do *not* spike your insulin. Therefore, how could they be dangerous?

They're dangerous for three reasons.

First, many people don't realize that glucose alone is not sweet to the taste, while fructose is. You can take anything, from cardboard to the cushion you're sitting on, dip it in HFCS, and it's delicious.

Second, fructose turns off the hormone leptin—the switch that tells you that you're satiated, satisfied. As a result, when you eat sugary fruit or cheesy corn curls packed with HFCS, your brain's satisfaction mechanism switches off. You don't stop until your stomach is literally physically full. And over time, your stomach dutifully accommodates by growing to stretch and increase capacity.

Third, and perhaps most important of all, fructose also stimulates a second hormone, ghrelin, which makes you feel hungry. When that happens, your stomach growls, you eat—probably a handy processed carbohydrate chocked full of HFCS and glucose. The cycle repeats itself over again. You are addicted. You know what

---

39 I had this conversation in the 1970s with a longtime friend and pediatrician. I argued that glucose and fructose sugars are different, and he disagreed. I didn't know the difference then, but intuitively I knew they *had* to be different.

you're doing is wrong, but it tastes so good and feels so satisfying that you eat the whole bag. Maybe you will stop at half a bag, but the true danger of fructose is that it keeps bringing you back to the sugar trough.

HFCS is designed to create fat. Just as bears preparing for a long hibernation gorge on berries filled with fructose, filling up every day on artificial food tells your body to put on fat as fast as possible. Eventually, you waddle out of McDonalds[40] to the doctor's office to be treated for some "-itis" or "-ectomy." It's really that simple. I know because I was once a waddler too—so much so that I had to have my gallbladder removed.

My pediatrician friend now has Alzheimer's, and his son, another pediatrician, studies autism. Sadly, as I'll discuss in later chapters, both are sugar-induced conformational diseases. I only wish we'd had the proof then that we do now.

WHAT ABOUT SUGAR SUBSTITUTES?

If HFCS is sugar's evil twin, then sugar substitutes are sugar's heartless doppelgänger. Heartless because artificial sweeteners are *not* a bridge to recovery—not the savior we were led to believe.

The World Health Organization warns against using acesulfame K, aspartame, advantame, cyclamates, neotame, saccharin, sucralose, stevia, and stevia derivatives as their long-term use puts you at greater risk for type 2 diabetes and heart disease.

---

40 It's important to note that because of recent public outrage, McDonalds removed HFCS from its sandwich buns, replacing it with just plain sugar. As the kids say, big whoop.

Several scholars have reported recently on a large study in France, concluding that consumption of sugar substitutes (especially aspartame, acesulfame potassium, and sucralose) is associated with increased risk of cardiovascular disease. A second study found that erythritol, a so-called natural sugar substitute, is also linked to cardiovascular disease.

In *Sugar Crush,* I rail on about artificial sweeteners at length, but let me mention two key points here. First, they are a crutch perpetuating the taste for sweetness. Few people know that the desire for sugar naturally subsides when you remove it from your diet (see chapter 7), while artificial sweeteners make withdrawal from sugar cravings harder, not easier. Second, artificial sweeteners (even stevia and allulose) not only lead to a rise in both insulin and blood glucose levels, but they're also detrimental to your essential gut flora—with long-term use causing symptoms of IBS and other gastric disorders. Avoid them.

THE FOES WHO OPPOSE

Meanwhile, scientists employed by manufacturers relying upon sugar still scramble to spin the evidence of sugar's destructive effects. In a recent *New York Times* editorial, Mike Blake with Reuters News Agency reported that when the mayor of Philadelphia sought to impose a tax on sugary beverages, one branch of the cola industry's trade group donated $10 million to the Children's Hospital of Philadelphia to study childhood obesity—while another division successfully lobbied the city council to kill the proposal.

Coca-Cola* has established an aggressive social media campaign touting its new mini can of Coke as a "beneficial" snack food while providing significant (sometimes "unrestricted") funding to prominent university researchers willing to tout the company's marketing strategy of shifting the focus of the obesity crisis from "sugary beverages" to "a need for more exercise."[41]

In the next chapter, I'll discuss other survival campaigns of the drug and artificial-food industries, along with the FDA's bumbling attempts to monitor sugar in our food chain.

---

41 I'm guessing their premise was that 100 calories from a Coke are the same as 100 calories from fudge, boiled chicken, broccoli, or whatever—and that exercise would offset one and all. This is simply false.

Bibliography

Abdelmalek, Manal F., Ayako Suzuki, Cynthia Guy, Aynur Unalp-Arida, Ryan Colvin, Richard J. Johnson, and Anna Mae Diehl. "Increased Fructose Consumption Is Associated with Fibrosis Severity in Patients with Nonalcoholic Fatty Liver Disease." *Hepatology* 51, no. 6 (2010): 1961–1971. https://doi.org/10.1002/hep.23535.

Abou-Donia, Mohamed B., Eman M. El-Masry, Ali A. Abdel-Rahman, Roger E. McLendon, and Susan S. Schiffman. "Splenda Alters Gut Microflora and Increases Intestinal P-Glycoprotein and Cytochrome P-450 in Male Rats." *Journal of Toxicology and Environmental Health, Part A: Current Issues* 71, no. 21 (2008): 1415–1429, https://doi.org/10.1080/15287390802328630.

Achim Burger, Leo, Stefan Stojkovic, André Diedrich, Svitlana Demyanets, Johann Wojta, and Thomas Pezawas. "Elevated Plasma Levels of Asymmetric Dimethylarginine and the Risk for Arrhythmic Death in Ischemic and Non-Ischemic, Dilated Cardiomyopathy—A Prospective, Controlled Long-Term Study." *Clinical Biochemistry* 83 (2020): 37–42. https://doi.org/10.1016/j.clinbiochem.2020.05.016.

Agrawal, Rahul, Emily Noble, Laurent Vergnes, Zhe Ying, Karen Reue, and Fernando Gomez-Pinilla. "Dietary Fructose Aggravates the Pathobiology of Traumatic Brain Injury by Influencing Energy Homeostasis and Plasticity." *Journal of Cerebral Blood Flow and Metabolism* 36, no. 5 (2016): 941–953. https://doi.org/10.1177/0271678X15606719.

Colt, Sam. "McDonald's Created Broccoli That Tastes Like Bubble Gum." *Business Insider*, November 14, 2014. https://www.businessinsider.com/mcdonalds-bubble-gum-broccoli-2014-11.

Cooke, John P. "ADMA: Its Role in Vascular Disease." *Society for Vascular Medicine* 10, no. S1 (2005): S11–S17. https://doi.org/10.1177/1358836X0501000103.

Cooke, John P. "Asymmetrical Dimethylarginine: The Uber Marker?" *Circulation* 109, no. 15 (2004): 1813–1818. https://doi.org/10.1161/01.CIR.0000126823.07732.D5.

Corliss, Julie. "Sugar Substitutes: New Cardiovascular Concerns?" Harvard Health Publishing. January 1, 2023. https://www.health.harvard.edu/heart-health/sugar-substitutes-new-cardiovascular-concerns.

Debras, Charlotte, Eloi Chazelas, Laury Sellem, Raphaël Porcher, Nathalie Druesne-Pecollo, Younes Esseddik, Fabien Szabo de Edelenyi, Cédric Agaësse, Alexandre De Sa, Rebecca Lutchia, Léopold K Fezeu, Chantal Julia, Emmanuelle Kesse-Guyot, Benjamin Allès, Pilar Galan, Serge Hercberg, Mélanie Deschasaux-Tanguy, Inge Huybrechts, Bernard Srour, and Mathilde Touvier. "Artificial Sweeteners and Risk of Cardiovascular Diseases: Results from the Prospective Nutrinet-Santé Cohort." *BMJ* 378 (2022). https://doi.org/10.1136/bmj-2022-071204.

Dellon, Arnold Lee, Susan E. Mackinnon, and W.A. Seiler. "Susceptibility of the Diabetic Nerve to Chronic Compression." *Annals of Plastic Surgery* 20, no. 2 (1988): 117–119. https://doi.org/10.1097/00000637-198802000-00004.

"Fructose Identified as Central Conduit to Obesity." News Medical Life Sciences. August 1, 2023. https://www.

news-medical.net/news/20230801/Fructose-identified-as-central-conduit-to-obesity.aspx.

Hayden, Melvin R. "Viremia and Interaction of Endothelial Cells, Erythrocytes, Leukocytes and Platelets in Type 2 Diabetes Mellitus and COVID-19: A Closer Look at Proposed Mechanisms." Preprint, submitted December 2020. https://doi.org/10.20944/preprints202012.0642.v1.

Horton, Mark, Philip Langton, and Alexander Bentley. "A History of Sugar—the Food Nobody Needs, but Everyone Craves." The Conversation. October 30, 2015. https://theconversation.com/a-history-of-sugar-the-food-nobody-needs-but-everyone-craves-49823.

"How Much Sugar Is Too Much?" Heart.org. Accessed April 14, 2024. https://www.heart.org/en/healthy-living/healthy-eating/eat-smart/sugar/how-much-sugar-is-too-much.

Jacoby, Richard P., and Raquel Baldelomar. *Sugar Crush: How to Reduce Inflammation, Reverse Nerve Damage, And Reclaim Good Health.* New York: Harper Wave, 2015.

Li, Xia, Weihua Li, Hong Wang, Douglas L. Bayley, Jie Cao, Danielle R. Reed, Alexander A. Bachmanov, Liquan Huang, Véronique Legrand-Defretin, Gary K. Beauchamp, and Joseph G. Brand. "Cats Lack a Sweet Taste Receptor." *The Journal of Nutrition.* 136, no. 7 (2006): 1932S–1934S. https://doi.org/10.1093/jn/136.7.1932S.

Liu, Jing, Caiying Li, Wen Chen, Kuanrong He, Huijuan Ma, Boqing Ma, Pei Zhao, and Lu Tian. "Relationship Between Serum Asymmetric Dimethylarginine Level and Microvascular Complications in Diabetes Mellitus: A Meta-Analysis." *BioMed Research International,* 2019: 2941861. https://doi.org/10.1155/2019/2941861.

Mayes, Susan Dickerson, and Hana Zickgraf. "Atypical Eating
   Behaviors in Children and Adolescents with Autism,
   ADHD, Other Disorders, and Typical Development."
   Research in Autism Spectrum Disorders 64 (2019): 76–83.
   https://doi.org/10.1016/j.rasd.2019.04.002.

"McDonalds Removes High Fructose Corn Syrup from Its
   Buns." WNAX. Accessed April 14, 2024. https://wnax.com/
   news/180081-mcdonalds-removes-high-fructose-corn-syrup-
   from-its-buns/.

Ming, Lee Chong. "CNA Explains: Are Sugar Substitutes Like
   Stevia and Saccharin Really Healthier?" CNA. Last updated
   May 24, 2023. https://www.channelnewsasia.com/singapore/
   non-sugar-sweeteners-artificial-substitute-safe-weight-loss-
   diabetes-calories-who-3494141.

Möckl, Leonhard. "The Emerging Role of the Mammalian
   Glycocalyx in Functional Membrane Organization and
   Immune System Regulation." *Frontiers in Cell and
   Development Biology* 8, no. 253 (2020): https://doi.org/
   10.3389/fcell.2020.00253.

The Editorial Board. "Coke Tries to Sugarcoat the Truth on
   Calories." *New York Times*, August 14, 2015. https://www.
   nytimes.com/2015/08/14/opinion/coke-tries-to-sugarcoat-
   the-truth-on-calories.html.

"Per Capita Sugar and Sweetener Consumption." IBIS World.
   October 18, 2023. https://www.ibisworld.com/us/bed/
   per-capita-sugar-sweetener-consumption/4669/.

Strong, Colby. "Serum ADMA Level as a Prognostic Biomarker
   for Amyotrophic Lateral Sclerosis." Neurology Advisor.
   March 3, 2022. https://www.neurologyadvisor.com/topics/
   neurodegenerative-diseases/serum-adma-level-prognostic-
   biomarker-amyotrophic-lateral-sclerosis/.

Tarkan, Laurie. "Big Soda in a Froth Over Proposed New Sugar-Labeling Rules." *Fortune*, July 29, 2015. https://www. fortune.com/2015/07/29/fda-nutrition-labels-sugar-soda/.

University of California San Francisco. "Hidden in Plain Sight." Sugar Science. Accessed April 14, 2024. https://sugarscience. ucsf.edu/hidden-in-plain-sight/.

Upton, Adrian R., and Alan J. McComas. "The Double Crush in Nerve-Entrapment Syndromes." *The Lancet* 2, no. 7825 (1973): 359–362. https://doi.org/10.1016/S0140-6736(73) 93196-6.

Wexler, Marisa. "Multiple Sclerosis Diet: Foods to Eat and Avoid." Multiple Sclerosis News Today. Last updated October 17, 2022. https://multiplesclerosisnewstoday.com/ living-with-ms/ms-diet-nutrition/healthy-eating-ms/.

"What You Need to Know About Allulose." Cleveland Clinic. August 25, 2022. https://health.clevelandclinic.org/what-is-allulose/amp.

Witkowski, Marco, Ina Nemet, Hassan Alamri, Jennifer Wilcox, Nilaksh Gupta, Nisreen Nimer, Arash Haghikia, Xinmin S. Li, Yuping Wu, Prasenjit Prasad Saha, Ilja Demuth, Maximilian König, Elisabeth Steinhagen-Thiessen, Tomas Cajka, Oliver Fiehn, Ulf Landmesser, W. H. Wilson Tang, and Stanley L. Hazen. "The Artificial Sweetener Erythritol and Cardiovascular Event Risk." *Nature Medicine* 29, no. 3 (2023): 710–718. https://doi.org/10.1038/s41591-023-02223-9.

CHAPTER 4

How We All Got Glued

—Big Pharma, big farming, and the artificial-food industry

It's difficult to get a man to understand something, when his salary depends on his not understanding it.

—Upton Sinclair[42]

Every successful drug ad seen on television follows a highly prescribed, polished script—and it uses pure Aristotelian logic to persuade.

Here's a typical drug ad:

FADE IN:

IMAGE. GORGEOUS SMALL-TOWN PARK, ANYWHERE, USA—DAY

---

42 Upton Sinclair, *I, Candidate for Governor and How I Got Licked by Upton Sinclair* (Berkley: University of California Press, 1934), 109.

A sunny day in the park. Enter relieved, SMILING PATIENT looking at [whatever our drug fixes].

SUPER: background, our jingle

SMILING PATIENT:

"I've been in the fight of my life with [insert disease],
and now with the help of [insert drug],
I'm living more of the life I deserve."

CONTINUOUS IMAGES:

Enter loved one(s) with baby or multiple grandchildren who run to Smiling Patient.

SUPER: amp up jingle

Smiling Patient begins dancing and is joined by wonderful new friends who just like her are moving forward, too, with their wonder drug. They comfort her for a bit, then laugh with one another and enjoy the day—as someone breaks out the picnic and lawn darts.

SUPER: chorus of our jingle,
drug name on screen
VOICE-OVER starts in mildly hushed tones

SPOKESPERSON VOICE-OVER
(fast-talking)
"Diarrhea and vomiting are common when taking [our drug]
also known as [insert generic equivalent] and may be severe.
Talk to your doctor if these symptoms persist."

CUT TO:

NEXT IMAGE. EVENING FADES TO NIGHT.

As the sun fades to darkness, Smiling Patient pauses to reflect. Picnic turns into full-blown barbeque party. Twinkle lights fill the trees. Clowns and jugglers entertain the smiling, dancing revelers. Someone gently brings Smiling Patient a cozy sweater, and she resumes enhanced life with her loved ones. Fireworks fill the night sky.

SUPER: fireworks explode, background
VOICE-OVER (the stuff they[43] make us say)

SPOKESPERSON VOICE-OVER
(softer and faster)
"In rare cases [our drug] has been known to cause serious liver problems, hair loss, infertility, blood clots, some cancers, and low white blood cell counts that can lead to death."

FADE OUT

---

43 It's the Federal Trade Commission (FTC) when our drug is over the counter, and it's the Food and Drug Administration (FDA) when our drug is a prescription.

Sometimes it seems that our entire health care system is out of whack—a ridiculous, perpetual movement of absurdities. For example, why do most physicians and the American Medical Association continue prescribing statin drugs when we know they cause serious long-term side effects including muscle damage, liver damage, peripheral neuropathy, increased blood sugar levels, memory loss or confusion, dizziness, depression, and weight gain? Especially when they don't even work on many people. A meta-analysis published by the British Medical Association reviewed the records of 164,411 patients and discovered that 51% had "failed to reach healthy cholesterol levels after two years [of statin treatment]."

Or how is it that drugs designed to relieve the symptoms of MS can literally cost patients tens of thousands of dollars per year? Even the American Diabetes Association—the organization dedicated to combating blood sugar levels—still tells its members to eat large quantities of sugar-laden grains, fruits, and vegetables.

For decades, we've been told that physicians weren't taught nutrition in school, but how long can this excuse hold water? The public is learning that sugar is bad and that eating keeps metabolism functioning. Why haven't our medical professionals learned? It's because it's in their best economic interest to do otherwise. Many well-intentioned physicians learn at what I call the University of Morton's—steakhouse, that is—wined and dined by pharmaceutical representatives who hand out perks to doctors who hand out pills to cover symptoms.

One study published by *JAMA* reported that even doctors who received a single, inexpensive meal (averaging less than $20, but a free meal from a Big Pharma rep nonetheless) were more likely to prescribe the brand-name medication being hawked. And as Marcia Angell, a former editor of the *New England Journal of Medicine*, says in her book *The Truth About the Drug Companies*, studies show that the morning after such Big Pharma dinners that company's sales can go up as high as 76%.

The last such dinner I attended was put on by Pfizer—at a very expensive restaurant complete with a $250 seafood pyramid group appetizer. That night they were pushing Lyrica® for the treatment of diabetic neuropathy (among its other uses). Besides a lavish appetizer designed to encourage mingling, such affairs always feature an expert speaker, and this time it was a neurologist and specialist in epilepsy who was from a prominent facility in a western state. Most of the drugs used in peripheral neuropathy are derivatives of drugs (such as Lyrica) that are commonly used by neurologists— and I'll give him credit because he certainly knew his drugs. The lecture was an interesting presentation on pharmacology from a historic perspective, and I certainly learned some things. However, he didn't know a thing about peripheral neuropathy. When he asked the audience for questions, I raised my hand.

"I notice that you didn't include Dr. Lee Dellon's theory of nerve compression."

What a firestorm that set off!

A LITTLE BACKSTORY

We doctors belong to separate disciplines, silos, or old boys' clubs— however you wish to frame it. Many specialists, neurologists and psychiatrists in particular, accept the *chemistry* of sugar inflammation, but they also think it only pertains to the brain, when, in fact, it pertains to every system, organ, and process in the body. And when I challenge their assumptions, it's as if I've *stepped on their nerves*, veered out of my lane and into theirs. At this particular University of Morton's gathering, mentioning Dellon was like celebrating the quarterback from a crosstown rival.

Dellon had been trained as a plastic surgeon, and early in his career, he took on a fellowship at the esteemed Curtis National Hand Center in Baltimore. He was already on the lowest rung of the ladder in this hierarchy of medicine, because if you talk to a neurologist, they own that domain. But in the mid- to late-1970s, our awareness of and procedures for carpal tunnel were just emerging. Surgeons at Curtis were developing seminal techniques and trying to figure out why, suddenly it seemed, people were developing excruciating and debilitating carpal tunnel syndrome.[44]

I understand the coincidence because back in those days, if I came across tarsal tunnel (which is the same thing in the foot—only a compression of the tibial nerve in the ankle), I'd refer the patient to a plastic surgeon to treat. I didn't yet have that skill set, and plastic surgery was then the specialty camp with the best or very good microsurgical techniques. Over time, the growing number of surgeries required for carpal tunnel moved into orthopedic surgery, which began dominating the field, with some doctors becoming exclusively hand surgeons. But then, in the 1980s and '90s, things took a sharp turn. The simple truth is that when plastic surgeons discovered the wonders of silicone, they'd ask

---

44 The time frame clearly corelates to the massive influx of HFCSs in the U.S. diet dominated by fast food.

themselves, Why would I operate on a peripheral nerve in the wrist for a few hundred dollars, when I can make $10 thousand for a reconstruction—and in the same amount of time? It became a matter of simple economics.

To his credit, Dr. Dellon stuck with it, perfecting his techniques, and eventually making the connection to compression as the culprit. Then, with more than 750 peer-reviewed articles and two textbooks on the topic, he crossed over into the neurologists' lane when he presented his compression theory of how sugar causes inflammation that compresses nerves and leads to all the diseases and conditions I call the "-itisis" and "-ectomies." His audacity was quickly followed by denunciation from none other than the world's leading authority in the world of neurology. A man I describe this way in my book *Sugar Crush:*

> Peter J. Dyck, of the Mayo Clinic in Rochester, Minnesota, is one of the leading neurologists in the country and author of a seminal two-volume textbook, *Peripheral Neuropathy* [which] dominates the neurology literature and thinking in the medical world. It is the gold standard for the accepted treatment of diabetic peripheral neuropathy, [then thought to be] an "incurable" disease.

When Dellon suggested use of his decompression techniques not only on carpal tunnel but on diabetic neuropathy of the foot and ankle, Dyck and the Mayo Clinic flipped out. How could this mere *plastic surgeon* tell neurologists how to do things? They sponsored a bulletin on the internet in which the American Neurological Association issued a warning that doing the Dellon decompression procedure was "too *dangerous* for high-risk diabetic patients." The grapevine made it up to Washington (specifically the Centers for Medicare & Medicaid Services) where it caused an absolute furor. Many years later, Dellon told me he had gone to the Mayo Clinic to discuss the bulletin directly with Dr. Dyck—who not only wouldn't discuss it but wouldn't even let Dellon into his office.

BACK AT THE SEAFOOD PYRAMID

After a few minutes of lively discussion on the pros and cons of prescription treatments and issues, the Lyrica representative jumped up. "Well, we're not here to talk about that. The FDA makes us stick to these slides that are preapproved."

Of course, I persisted, and turning to the speaker said, "I can understand that, but I'd still like to hear your comments."

"No, I really can't comment on that," the neurologist said.

I looked to the physicians sitting at my table, and they were squirming in their seats. My colleagues were afraid to speak up. They didn't want to hear that medication was just a short-term fix. They didn't want to hear how a simple procedure could relieve the pain of neuropathy because they weren't surgeons, and they couldn't do it. All they had were the gifts from our host (leather-bound pads and matching pens) with which to write prescriptions for Lyrica or the generic gabapentin—which simply dulls the pain. Besides, *not* writing those prescriptions and *fixing* the problem instead would mean lost revenue.

Pfizer was paying for our dinner, and I was suddenly the awkward guest making a scene—sneezing on the seafood, if you will.

So, I turned to the gathering and said, "Okay, I'll shut up because I want all you guys to get dessert."

These dinners take place every night hundreds, if not thousands, of times across the country. How do such events affect patients? Well, let's look back to Keith, the patient with MS you met in chapter 3, and to the Zamboni procedure, which has relieved the symptoms of tens of thousands of MS patients around the world.[45]

For years, Keith had been prescribed 800 mg of Neurontin (gabapentin) three times a day with a chaser of Voltaren. No one ever told him about Dellon's nerve-compression technique or Zamboni's process—which would have at least eased his pain without drugs.

And no doctor certainly ever told Keith to simply stop eating sugar. Meanwhile, drugs to relieve the symptoms of MS can literally cost patients like Keith $100 thousand per year—which lines a lot of pockets in the realm of Big Pharma. Most patients are kept happy because insurance (including Medicare and Medicaid) pays the bill, and the pain goes away—a Pyrrhic victory because the drug works to dull the brain while doing nothing to stop the ongoing damage.

Still, if I'm a pharmaceutical rep, I'm going to wine and dine physicians to gently persuade them to prescribe my drug of record. And I'm certainly going to discourage them from ever talking to some crackpot podiatrist with a simple theory. Predictably, I don't get invited to many such dinners anymore.

45 Angioplasty to dilate the jugular vein thus relieving the patient's vagus nerve. In 2017, Zamboni himself conceded that his procedure did not *cure* MS. That's because the cure is to un-glue the nerves, not relieve venous blood flow from the brain to the heart.

I'M NOT AGAINST PHARMACEUTICALS

I accept that in a free-market society, pharmaceuticals are hocked on TV like cheap tube socks. As comedian Bill Maher noted, "When you tell your doctor [what pills are right for you], isn't he just a dealer at that point?" So, is it any wonder we pop *whatever pill* to just help *whatever*? You and your grandchildren can probably sing several jaunty little drug jingles.

And yet when we need drugs—we *really* need them.

Needing them doesn't mean we should stop being vigilant, though. For example, let's take something simple like antibiotics, which have proven to be highly effective go-to drugs. It's happened more than once: yellow fever, gonorrhea,[46] meningitis, pneumonia, acne—you get the point. No doubt, if you are in a public park and get bitten by a squirrel with the plague—or more likely, a flea off a squirrel with the plague—you will want a great, big dose of antibiotics. As well you should. It's not hyperbole to say that antibiotics have saved humanity, more than once. And we count on them to do so again when necessary.

And yet, we must also discuss how some errant, little bugs have survived the warrior antibiotics, grown stronger, and are now coming back for revenge. It's called antibiotic resistance, and even more frightening is that researchers at the University of London discovered that bacteria share genetic material through their cell walls, thus "teaching" one another how to resist our best efforts

---

46 Although antibiotics once cured gonorrhea, the CDC reports indicate that a painful antibiotic-resistant gonorrhea is on the increase, especially among people in the 15–24 age range.

to eradicate them. Their success rate is staggering, as each year, more than 2.8 million Americans become infected with bacteria resistant to antibiotics, resulting in an estimated 35,000 deaths annually. One infection in particular, *Clostridioides difficile* (nickname, C. diff.), causes a deadly diarrhea that, according to the Centers for Disease Control and Prevention, accounts for nearly 13,000 of those deaths per year. Most of those deaths occur among the very young and the very old.

No, I'm not against pharmaceuticals. I'm against the fact they're priced too high. I'm against the fact that Big Pharma controls both the prices and the research because Big Pharma also controls the academic institutions conducting that research. The connection is no better documented than in the previously mentioned book by Marcia Angell in which she says, in part, that "drug companies often contract with academic researchers to carry out studies for almost entirely commercial purposes." And these same companies "are given virtually unfettered access to young doctors to ply them with gifts and meals and promote their wares." She calls the last practice "marketing masquerading as education."

We're stuck between a rock and a hard place, as the saying goes. Our system of governance is designed to accept the opinions of all when making the laws that govern us all. That's the theory. And at best it means your vote and your call to your elected representative will make an impact on their decision. At worst it means big-money lobbyists—a.k.a., Big Pharma (and the like)—literally write the legislation protecting them and their profits. In addition, medical researchers "employed" by Big Pharma naturally rise within the ranks of our federal oversight programs.

One recent example involves the naming of Dr. Monica Bertagnolli as the 16th director of the National Institutes of Health, who while serving at prestigious hospitals and medical societies also received 116 grants (worth $290.8 million) from Pfizer. Robert F. Kennedy Jr. has tweeted "Does this mean Dr. Bertagnolli is personally corrupt? Not at all. But it does mean that she will probably represent the viewpoints and priorities of the pharmaceutical industry. This is how agencies are captured."

In 2021, the U.S. House Committee on Oversight and Reform reported on a three-year investigation after which Chair Carol B. Maloney (D-NY) announced that Big Pharma's pricing practices are "unsustainable, unjustifiable, and unfair." For example, the committee found that the 12 best-selling drugs in Medicare are now "priced at a median of almost 500% higher than when they were brought to market."

Higher prices are always cited as the cost of high-quality R&D, yet the committee also found that over a five-year period, while the top 14 drug companies spent billions on research and development, much of that money was dedicated to finding ways to extend patent protections and anticompetitive strategies (not to mention slick TV commercials). During that same period, $577 million had been spent on stock buybacks and dividends to stockholders.

I like stock dividends; I'm not even opposed to someone buying me a dinner. But when it's by pharm reps, it feels like bribery. If someone spends $100 on my dinner—more if I like the expensive bourbon—then I must accept that person wants something. And when I question my hosts, they tell me to shut up, as if to say, "I'm buying the dinner, and I'm buying you." In the current scheme of things, any treatment or procedure not falling in lockstep with the system is shuffled off to Buffalo, deep-sixed, or simply legislated out of existence by the big boys.

That's why I sincerely believe that every patient must recognize that you're *not* entering the health care system for "*health* care," because most physicians, hospitals, and the companies big enough to buy all those dinners are not in the health care business. They are in the *pathology repair business*. The only good news is that once you're *un*-glued, you won't need the medicines that have been merely masking your symptoms.

So, maybe what I'm most against is how the avarice of the pharmaceutical industry has leached into our food chain.

BIG PHARMA MEETS BIG FARMING—A.K.A. THE RISE OF THE ARTIFICIAL-FOOD INDUSTRY

According to Fortune Business Insights: "The U.S. pharmacy market is projected to grow from $560 billion[47] in 2021 to $861.67 billion by 2028." And according to sources such as the nonprofit Natural Resources Defense Council, an estimated 70% of all antibiotics sold in the U.S. are used in the food and water of industrial livestock—primarily pigs, cattle, and chickens. While the obvious motivation is to increase yield (animals growing bigger, faster), antibiotics are also used as a prophylactic to compensate for unhealthy living conditions.

---

47 $200 billion of that astronomical amount is attributed to the sales of one drug, Humira—the immunosuppressive prescribed most often for arthritis, plaque psoriasis, ankylosing spondylitis, Crohn's disease, and ulcerative colitis. The average cost without insurance (and using an online coupon) is $6,240 for a two-pen box.

In other words, industrial producers try to inoculate against their livestock living in cramped, squalid conditions in hopes most of the "product" will fend off the unhealthy bacteria they wallow in. Upon entering the food chain, the drug-resistant bacteria that develop in these environments are superpredators and account for most of the antibiotic resistance seen in humans.

We have depleted our natural food chain. We no longer grow our own organic food, relying instead upon overly processed, hormone-injected, and artificial "food substitutes." As a result, a single shrimp with a suspect gut in a poorly run Thai fish farm can easily enter your food chain or those of your children. Whole grain from wholesome Iowa or California farmers trying to protect the heritage of their grandchildren throws your gut cells for a loop because of what those farmers must do to bring you the cheap, plentiful food you've come to expect—out of season and in perfect cosmetic beauty—just like the photo spreads in the best cookbooks. When's the last time you bought an oblong peach? Or a zucchini that had matured on the ground? Modern soil differs significantly from that which fed our ancestors just 100 years ago. And meanwhile, we've brought plant species "in from the wild," adapting them to "unorthodox" (i.e., more profitable) climatic zones and aesthetics—all for the glory of the varietal marketplace.

Modern agriculture began in the late 18th to early 19th centuries with something prophetically called the Malthusian catastrophe. Like others of his era, the right Reverend Robert Thomas Malthus, a British cleric and social activist, was horrified by what he saw in the slums of London: too many people and too little food. Not only that, but the soil was dead throughout the breadbaskets of Europe. Crops were puny, and demand had depleted God's bounty.

Malthus and his followers concluded that they had come to the end of civilization. And so, a century later, this prevailing social zeitgeist led scientist Fritz Haber to place atmospheric nitrogen under high temperature and create fertilizer, which in 1918 earned him the Nobel Prize for Chemistry.[48] The kicker was that over the long term—just about now—we discovered that nitrogen fertilizer was not exactly what plant biology requires for natural development.

Specifically, this new nitrogen fertilizer chemically bonds to a plant's root system, travels up the root stem, becomes intimately involved in photosynthesis, and enters the plant's cellular structure. Eating any chemical that such plants have "ingested" means real-time consequences for the health of your own gut biome.

We're Just Getting Started

Nitrogen fertilizer is just the start because it's usually combined with the herbicide, glyphosate—the primary ingredient in Monsanto's herbicide RoundUp" (originally used for weed control).

Efforts to have glyphosate removed from our food chain were thwarted when a rider to the Senate Continuing Resolution spending bill, HR 933.1, Section 735 (dubbed the Monsanto Protection Act) was slipped through Congress when most of us weren't looking. In this rider (passed during the sequestration of 2013), Monsanto is protected against any future legal action regarding the side effects of its herbicides, seeds, or GMO crops.

---

48 Haber also developed the infamous chemical warfare program Germany launched in WWI.

Oregon has banned glyphosate for more than 30 years. Other states and individual cities have followed with warnings and specific restrictions such as banning use on playgrounds or public walkways. A full 28 nations around the world ban it outright, and yet, before Russia's attack on Ukraine, John Deere and Monsanto were introducing glyphosate into Ukraine, the breadbasket of Europe.

Meanwhile, new science tells us that glyphosate in combination with aluminum (used in the new aerial-spraying protocols) leads to disease in the pineal gland. That consequence in turn is linked to destruction of the gut microbiome and neurological disease. And in 2015, the International Agency for Research on Cancer (part of the World Health Organization) labeled glyphosate as "probably carcinogenic" for consumers.

The coincidence is relevant because, through a complex biochemical reaction (the nitric oxide pathway) discussed in *Sugar Crush*, glyphosate increases vasoconstriction (the narrowing of tiny blood vessels), a major contributor to how we all get glued.

Since 1972 when we first started taking notice, corn has remained the top pesticide-drenched crop in the country.[49] At the same time, the most recent (2019) data gathered tells us that the per capita consumption of corn products is 336.5 pounds a year.[50] That's not just on the cob and out of the can but includes flour and meal, hominy and grits, and food starch additives in artificial food.

---

49 Soybeans are number two.
50 Just to keep things in focus, remember the formula used in an earlier chapter: carbohydrate grams divided by four equals the number of teaspoons of sugar. One medium ear full of fresh sweet corn has approximately 41 grams of carbohydrates. That's **10.25 teaspoons of sugar**. (You *need* but one teaspoon of added sugar per day to keep your metabolism humming.)

And corn is high in the unhealthy omega-6 fatty acids that promote inflammation. For a brilliant and detailed analysis of how and why we consume so much corn, I'll direct you to "Corn: The Welfare Crop," an essay by scientist Micha Petty covering "the environmental and economic travesty of subsidized crops." In it, he tells us that corn subsidies (that means your tax dollars) in the U.S. between 1995 and 2019 totaled $113.9 billion, producing 75 billion cubic feet of corn. Or as he translates that volume, 821 piles of corn, each the size of the Great Pyramid of Giza. Perry concludes we have so much corn in large part because of government subsidies that foster overproduction, which artificially lowers prices, which leads to more corn in our food supply because it's cheap filler for food (not to mention dependency on its use in unleaded gasoline).

WHERE ARE OUR PROTECTORS?

Who protects us from the industrialization of sugar? Most Americans assume there is a federal agency protecting the nation's food supply, but unfortunately a more accurate appraisal is that such would-be protectors are missing in action. In 2022, in a wonderful evaluation of the long-term inadequacies of the Food and Drug Administration, *Politico* detailed the agency's abysmal history of allowing deadly contaminated foods to slip through the net, as well as neglectfully slow recalls for everything from *E. coli* in packaged "leafy greens" to heavy metals and arsenic in baby food. *Politico* specifically cited the Center for Food Safety and Applied Nutrition, which is the FDA division charged with ensuring that the food you buy is free from harmful contaminants. The report concludes, "The division suffers from a deep-seated culture of avoiding hard decisions and a near-paralyzing fear of picking serious fights with the food industry." The agency has also failed to enact a 2011 safety reform bill designed to keep deadly pathogens out of the water used for agriculture.

And things aren't looking up for the regulators. During the eight-month period from October 1, 2022, to June 1, 2023, 230 regulators retired from the CFSAN staff of approximately 18,000—adding to the more than 2,000 current vacancies.

It's unfortunate, but the romantic Norman Rockwell depiction of farm life in America is rare. Today's commercial farms are far less likely to be governed by traditional, organic/ecological practices and more likely to be controlled by large corporations, which are driven only by maximizing profits and improving quarterly results and stock prices. This short-term thinking has left us with chemically contaminated soil, water, plants, and animals.

That horror brings us back to sugar, and specifically HFCS, the cheap food filler made from corn poisoned with herbicides like glyphosate. Everything in the grocery store is filled with sugar—even most of the meat. That's because most cows being prepared for food supply are fed corn. That's not their normal diet. Left to their own devices, cows will eat primarily grass.[51] But pent up and fed nothing but corn (which because of its high glucose content will fatten them up more quickly), cows will eat corn. The result is that glucose permeates their muscle tissue, producing a very toxic omega-6 fatty acid that winds up in our grocery carts and our bodies.

The poster child for how we all got glued is a well-produced contrivance called breakfast cereal. This brilliant marketing ploy to

---

51 Along with legumes, alfalfa, clover, hay, and occasionally foraged fruit.

sell corn and oats as "natural carbohydrate sugars" is made complete with added sucrose and fructose (to enhance the bland taste of grain). And as a result, young parents learned to soothe babies and placate toddlers with little baggies of cereal whenever adults must tend to business. I'm surprised they didn't calm Prince Louis at his grandfather's coronation with a little baggie of Fruit Loops.[52]

To wrap it up, we are surrounded by artificial food filled with sugar—which is poison and causes most diseases. But as a society we seem stuck with what we've got because sugar is so addictive, profitable, and thus encouraged by Big Pharma, Big Farming, and the federal regulatory system, which is supposed to be our big protector—but isn't. The path loops back to doctors and drugs to solve that equation—but they don't.

I'll admit it's starting to sound a little grim. Not to fear, because if you believe in the science of evolution, Lucy, our common *Homo sapiens* ancestor of 3.2 million years ago, passed along to us a magical substance that treats just about any inflammatory disease. I'm speaking of human growth cells—the solvent to *un*-glue and regenerate—and is the topic of the next three chapters.

---

52 Too much sugar mainly from breakfast cereal also fosters constant ear infections as well, but it's unlikely an ENT physician will tell you that.

Bibliography

Akyea, Ralph Kwame, Joe Kai, Nadeem Qureshi, Barbara Iyen, and Stephen F. Weng. "Sub-Optimal Cholesterol Response to Initiation of Statins and Future Risk of Cardiovascular Disease." *Heart* 105, no. 13 (2019): 975–981. https://doi.org/10.1136/heartjnl-2018-314253.

Angell, Marcia. *The Truth About the Drug Companies: How They Deceive Us and What to Do About It.* New York: Random House, 2005.

Aronson, Lauren. "Congress Must Meet the Moment to Hold Big Pharma Accountable." *Congress Blog.* Hill. December 28, 21. https://thehill.com/blogs/congress-blog/healthcare/587562-congress-must-meet-the-moment-to-hold-big-pharma-accountable.

Branswell, Helen. "Scientist Concedes His Controversial MS Therapy, Once a Source of Great Hope, Is 'Largely Ineffective.'" Stat. November 28, 2017. https://www.statnews.com/2017/11/28/multiple-sclerosis-paolo-zamboni/.

Brook, Lena. "To Protect the Future, Protect Antibiotics." Food, Farm Animals, and Drugs, Natural Resources Defense Council. May 18, 2020. www.nrdc.org/food/saving-antibiotics.asp.

Centers for Disease Control and Prevention. "Antibiotic Resistance Threats in the United States 2019." Centers for Disease Control and Prevention. Accessed April 15, 2024. https://www.cdc.gov/drugresistance/pdf/threats-report/2019-ar-threats-report-508.pdf.

Costa, Tiago, Catarina Felisberto-Rodrigues, Amit Meir, Marie S Prevost, Adam Redzej, Martina Trokter, and Gabriel

Waksman. "Secretion Systems in Gram-Negative Bacteria: Structural and Mechanistic Insights." *Nature Reviews/ Microbiology* 13 no. 6 (2015): 343–359. https://doi.org/10.1038/nrmicro3456.

Curry, Melanie. "Can You Eat Corn if You're on the Keto Diet?" *Men's Health*, July 6, 2021. https://www.menshealth.com/nutrition/a36792963/is-corn-keto/.

DeJong, Colette, Thomas Aguillar, Chien-Wen Tseng, Grace A. Lin, W. John Boscardin, and R. Adams Dudley. "Pharmaceutical Industry-Sponsored Meals and Physicians Prescribing Patterns for Medicare Beneficiaries." *JAMA Internal Medicine* 176, no. 8 (2016): 1114–1122. https://doi.org/10.1001/jamainternmed.2016.2765.

Dyck, Peter J., P. James B. Dyck, Christopher J. Klein, Phillip A. Low, Kimberly Amrami, JaNean Engelstad, and Robert J. Spinner. *Companion to Peripheral Neuropathy: Illustrated Cases and New Developments.* Philadelphia: Saunders, 2010.

Evich, Helena Bottemiller. "The FDA's Food Failure." *Politico*, April 8, 2022. https://www.politico.com/interactives/2022/fda-fails-regulate-food-health-safety-hazards.

Fallon, Sally, and Mary G. Enig. "Dangers of Statin Drugs: What You Haven't Been Told About Popular Cholesterol-Lowering Medicines." The Weston A. Price Foundation. July 14, 2004. https://www.westonaprice.org/health-topics/modern-diseases/dangers-of-statin-drugs-what-you-havent-been-told-about-popular-cholesterol-lowering-medicines/.

Goldberg, Elyssa. "How the U.S. Military Is Infiltrating Your Kitchen." *Bon Appétit*, July 15, 2015. https://www.bonappetit.com/entertaining-style/pop-culture/article/military-food.

Goldstein, Amy. "House Democrats Find in Three-Year
    Investigation That Drug Prices Are 'Unsustainable,
    Unjustifiable and Unfair.'" *Washington Post*, last updated
    December 10, 2021. https://www.washingtonpost.com/
    health/2021/12/10/house-democrats-find-three-year-inves-
    tigation-that-drug-prices-are-unsustainable-unjustifiable-
    unfair/.

"The Haber Process Nitrogen Fertilizer from the Air." The
    Compost Gardener.com. Accessed April 15, 2024. www.the-
    compost-gardener.com/haber-process.html.

Hoff, Mary. "The Case of Too Much or Too Little Nitrogen
    Fertilizer." University of Minnesota. April 17, 2013.

"How Much Does Humira Cost Without Insurance?" Drugs.
    com. Last updated April 4, 2024. https://www.drugs.com/
    medical-answers/humira-cost-without-insurance-3537595/.

Kanchwala, Hussain. "Malthusian Catastrophe: Will We Fall
    Short of Food Sources Due to Population Explosion?"
    ScienceABC. Last updated October 19, 2023. https://www.
    scienceabc.com/humans/malthusian-catastrophe-shortage-of-
    food-sources-population-explosion.html.

Kennedy, Robert F. Jr. (@RobertKennedyJr). "Does this mean
    Dr. Bertagnolli is personally corrupt? Not at all. But it
    does mean that she will probably represent the viewpoints
    and priorities of the pharmaceutical industry…" Twitter,
    May 16, 2023. https://twitter.com/RobertKennedyJr/
    status/1658476107996495878.

King, Gilbert. "Fritz Haber's Experiments in Life and Death."
    Smithsonian, June 6, 2012. https://www.smithsonianmag
    .com/history/fritz-habers-experiments-in-life-and-death-
    114161301/.

Landrigan, Phillip J., and Charles Benbrook. "GMOs, Herbicides,
and Public Health." *New England Journal of Medicine* 373, no. 8
(2015): 693–695. https://doi.org/10.1056/NEJMp1505660.

Morgan, Kendall K. "High Cholesterol: When Statins Don't
Work." WebMD. July 18, 2023. https://www.webmd.com/
cholesterol-management/cholesterol-tests-statin-resistant.

Perry, Micha. "Corn: The Welfare Crop." *The Natural World*
(blog). Medium. September 21, 2019. https://medium.com/
natural-world/corn-the-welfare-crop-ff7b053890ea.

Samsel, Anthony, and Stephanie Seneff. "Glyphosate's
Suppression of Cytochrome P450 Enzymes and Amino Acid
Biosynthesis by the Gut Microbiome: Pathways to Modern
Diseases." *Entropy* 15, no. 4 (2013): 1416–1463. https://doi.
org/10.3390/e15041416.

"The U.S. Pharmacy Market Is Projected to Grow From $560.00
Billion in 2021 to $861.67 Billion by 2028 at a CAGR Of
6.3% in Forecast Period, 2021–2028…" Fortune Business
Insights. January 28, 2022. https://www.fortunebusinessin-
sights.com/u-s-pharmacy-market-106306.

"A View from Congress: Role of Pharmacy Benefit Managers
in Pharmaceutical Markets." Committee on Oversight and
Reform. December 10, 2021. https://oversight.house.gov/
wp-content/uploads/2021/12/PBM-Report-12102021.pdf.

"Where Is Glyphosate Banned?" Wisner Baum. Last updated
May 2023. https://www.wisnerbaum.com/toxic-tort-law/
monsanto-roundup-lawsuit/where-is-glyphosate-banned.

"Who Is Really in Charge of America's Health?" CNN
Transcripts. August 5, 2004. https://transcripts.cnn.com/
show/pzn/date/2004-08-05/segment/00.

Wilkerson, John. "More Than 200 FDA Staffers Have Retired in Less Than a Year." Stat. June 6, 2023. https://www.statnews.com/2023/06/06/fda-retirements/.

Wunsch, Nils-Gerrit. "Per Capita Consumption of Corn Products in the US 2000–2019." Statista. June 1, 2022. https://www.statista.com/statistics/184202/per-capita-consumption-of-corn-products-in-the-us-since-2000.

PART II
Stem Cells

CHAPTER 5

Células Madre

—the solvent that un-glues your cells

Several months ago, Jim, an anesthesiologist, friend, and colleague, was desperate to relieve the intermittent symptoms that were confounding him and his doctors. The signs started off as severe headaches, fatigue, and systemic pain—and then progressed to intermittent aphasia.[53]

Jim's been a dedicated athlete his entire life—an avid skier, plus a national ranking in tennis. Like many Americans, he felt that if he exercised and stayed in shape, he could eat whatever he wanted. So, he loaded up on "heart-healthy" carbs—never equating stacks of pancakes, pasta, hearty oatmeal, or orange-mango smoothies[54] with sugar. I can understand such reasoning, because before my sugar epiphany I was *just like that*. I went to the gym every day.

---

53 Sometimes occurring after a stroke or head injury, aphasia is damage to the part of the brain that controls language expression (speech) and comprehension.

54 Making matters worse, insulin literally blocks vitamin C from entering your cells when glucose is present. (The molecules are separated by only two carbon atoms.) Acting like a bouncer at the club door, insulin allows glucose in, while vitamin C gets washed out through your excretory system.

I stayed in shape, and like Jim, I ate what we'd all been told to eat to stay healthy—the food pyramid, with 6 to 11 servings of carbohydrates as its base.

I was also an early adapter of regenerative therapies, confident they were safe and effective, while very carefully trying to determine correct doses to help my patients. However, a most revelatory experience came in 2016 when I experienced my own herniated disc. I went immediately to the neurologist and for a year thereafter did whatever I could to find a nonsurgical solution. Epidurals, acupuncture, physical therapy, ice packs, Advil, hanging upside down—you name it, I did it, including a trip to a pain center. Nothing worked. It was horrible.

One day I said to my neurosurgeon, "You know, I've been using amnionic fluid and umbilical cord tissue for lots of different inflammatory diseases in my practice. Why don't we try that on my back?"

"There's not enough research," he said with skepticism.

"I get that," I said. "But my only other option is surgery. What's the risk of just *trying* stem cells first? If they don't work, we can always take the surgery route."

He wasn't convinced. So, I left his office, went upstairs to my own, and prepared an injection of umbilical cord tissue.

I asked the naturopath who worked in my practice, "If I mark the spot, will you give it to me?"

"Sure."

That was a Wednesday. Friday, I didn't feel much better, so I called the neurosurgeon and scheduled a microdiscectomy. The next morning, I was in my kitchen having coffee when a friend called asking why he hadn't seen me at tennis. I started explaining about my disc, put my hand on the small of my back and suddenly realized that I had no pain. None. That was it. One shot—and I was back playing tennis in three days. I haven't felt that disc since. Meanwhile, I've also had regenerative therapy for shoulder pain and a ripped plantaris tendon.[55] I'm a believer. I know that it works.

So, when my friend Jim told me of his desperation and how he couldn't find a physician to either fully diagnose or treat him, I suggested he go to Neil Riordan's Stem Cell Institute in Panama.

We Americans are arrogant when proclaiming we have the best medicine in the world. Selling drugs, yes. Performing surgeries, yes. But if you want to become healthy—or recover quickly and efficiently from disease, injury, or even from simple surgery—well, then, no. To do that, you may need to travel to a place like Panama. And if you're set on getting world-class regenerative stem cell treatment[56] you may seek out Riordan's clinic on the gleaming, sunlit 75th floor of a Panama City high-rise. One point to further establish the context: Noriega is long gone, and the political situation currently is stable.

---

55   My patients with torn plantaris tendons often come in asking me to look for a bullet hole. It's that painful, as if you've been shot in the leg. Believe me, it will drop you to your knees.

56   Using biology, chemistry, medicine, computer sciences, robotics, genetics, engineering, and medicine to replace or regenerate cells, tissues, or organs to restore normal function.

Riordan is not a physician; he is a physician assistant and PhD in health sciences from the Medical University of the Americas. He has made several novel discoveries in the field of cancer research since the mid-1990s when he collaborated with his father, Dr. Hugh Riordan, on the effects of high-dose intravenous vitamin C on cancer cells and the tumor microenvironment. This pioneering study on vitamin C's preferential toxicity to cancer cells notably led to a 1997 patent for the treatment of cancer with vitamin C. In 2010, Dr. Riordan was granted an additional patent for a new cellular vaccine for cancer patients. Established in 2006, his Stem Cell Institute is one of the oldest, most well-known, and most well-respected stem cell therapy clinics in the world.

Jim couldn't walk well enough to make the trip alone, so I offered to go with him to lend support. During a layover in Houston, I called John Cooke, MD, PhD, (who was introduced in chapter 1) formerly with Stanford, who's now the director and chief investigator for inducible pluripotent stem cell research at Houston Methodist Hospital. John's one of the world's leading cardiologists and vascular biologists. His latest paper recently came out, and he congratulated me on being right about the effect that ADMA has in the constriction of blood vessels.

I laughed. "Yeah, it only took the rest of you guys fifteen years to figure that out."

The public is getting mixed messages about regenerative therapies, but the real researchers know that it works. My neurosurgeon was right, by the way, in his statement that there isn't enough research—*why* that's true will be an important point in chapter 5. But I'm getting ahead of myself.

STEM CELLS: WHAT THEY ARE AND WHAT THEY AREN'T

If you've neither had nor known someone who has had regenerative therapies, you might believe the common misperception that stem cells exist only in developing human embryos. It's true that during fetal development (gestation), stem cells evolve into every other kind of human cell, but after we're born, we each retain a limited reserve of stem cells stored in various parts of our bodies (primarily in bone marrow). These specialized cells are at the ready when needed to regenerate or repair tissues and organs.

As of this writing, there are four general categories of stem cells:

- **Embryonic stem cells.** Taken from donated embryos three to five days old (known during this period as a blastocyst and consisting of approximately 150 cells). Embryonic stem cells are pluripotent in that they can develop into any type of cell (such as nerve, bone, blood, skin, etc.). Thus, when injected into a diseased organ or damaged tissue, they can stimulate repair and regeneration of the patient's own tissue and organs.
- **Adult stem cells.** The word "adult" can be misleading because they also reside in infants, children, and cadavers. (I recognize those three create an awkward juxtaposition.) Rather, the term means that having done their pluripotent job of creating any type of cell, stem cells seemed to early researchers to settle down as site-specific cell types (blood, nerve, bone, etc.). They congregate primarily in bone marrow but also (in small numbers) at various sites such as skin, fat, and even hair follicles.

The most well-known adult stem cell therapy is probably the use of stem cells found in a patient's own bone marrow to marshal the fight against blood-cancer cells.

- **Altered adult stem cells.** Emerging technologies involve altering genes in adult cells so that they react more like embryonic stem cells. For example, scientists can now trigger bone marrow cells to give rise not only to blood cells but to bone or muscle cells as well. In addition, connective tissue stem cells have been "reprogrammed" into functional heart cells providing improved heart function and patient survival time.

- **Perinatal stem cells.** Sometimes also referred to as an adult cell, these are the stem cells found in perinatal *tissue*. This tissue would be otherwise discarded umbilical cord and placental tissues—especially Wharton's jelly, the rich, gelatinous substance within the umbilical cord.

  Perinatal stem cells are superior to other adult stem cells because they're immunologically privileged, meaning there is no antigen-antibody reaction. This has developed because, biologically speaking, a fetus in utero is a body foreign to the mother. So nature prevents her antibodies from going on the attack. Having no antigen-antibody reaction means there is little to no chance of cell rejection.

  Perinatal tissue (as well as the amnionic fluid bathing the fetus) is also full of **growth factors** (specialized proteins), which while not technically stem cells, nevertheless stimulate the growth and efficacy of stem cells. More on this later.

Your own innate stem cells are working this very minute (efficiently or inefficiently) in the ongoing process of repairing and/or regenerating specialized cells throughout your body. For example, cells in the small intestine are renewed every two to four days; the skin, every two weeks; and skeletal cells, every 10 years. Stem cells are the fundamental triggers in this natural healing/regenerative process.

How Do Stem Cells Heal Anyway?

You probably learned in seventh-grade health class that as a first step in healing, your body makes antibodies to fight off infection. Stem cells are key to this process. Once triggered, they cause a reaction in your immune system that blocks inflammation and facilitates the acceleration of tissue repair. The older the cells, the slower the process—and you've undoubtedly observed the effect in action. A tiny cut made by a baby's own fingernail on his opposite hand can heal in a matter of hours. Depending upon your general state of health, a tiny paper cut on your own hand can take a week or 10 days to heal.

A Deeper Dive

Once the mechanism was understood, it didn't take long for researchers to learn how to harness adult stem cells and use them for therapeutic purposes—fighting infection (most notably early on with skin grafts), easing the pain and dysfunction associated with diseases such as MS and arthritis and rallying the body's immune system to fight invading cancer cells.

The important point is that in the U.S., use of *embryonic* stem cells is highly restricted. In some states, researchers may only use embryonic stem cells donated after in vitro fertilization. Use of embryonic stem cells for regenerative therapy is illegal in the U.S.

However, they can be legally obtained and used for therapeutic purposes in other parts of the world, including Greece, the U.K., Sweden, Spain, and the Netherlands. And until the Russian invasion, Kiev was the site of one of the world's premier embryonic stem cell research facilities, the Academy of Medical Sciences of Ukraine. In the U.S., we may use cells that are harvested from an individual's own stem cell reserves, or we may use nonembryonic adult stem cells.

When considering stem cell therapies in the U.S., the question becomes "Are you really getting stem cells after all?" The uncertainty is because in the harvesting process of being frozen and preserved, they die. And if they're not alive, they're technically not stem cells. What the pioneer scientists are learning—and chief among them is Arnold Caplan, PhD—is that stem cells aren't what's doing the work anyway—it's the *growth factors*. Approximately 500 different kinds of growth factors have been identified so far, but that's deeper than we need to go on our first dive.

Caplan also refined the nomenclature of stem cells by coining the phrase "mesenchymal[57] stem cells" (now known throughout the medical lexicon as MSC). Several years later, after more experience with the subject (and being smart enough to realize he'd never be able to change the acronym), he proposed a name change from mesenchymal stem cells to medicinal signaling cells "to more accurately reflect the fact that these cells home in on sites of injury or disease and secrete bioactive factors that are immunomodulatory and tropic (regenerative)." The discovery means that a patient's

---

57 A word meaning undifferentiated, mostly mesodermal (in the middle layer) cells, which comprise connective tissues, blood, lymphatics, bone, and cartilage.

own "tissue-specific resident stem cells" are doing the actual work of reconstruction and repair.

How does that happen?

The Microuniverse of Pericytes, Exosomes, and Growth Factors

When you take a pain killer—let's say basic aspirin—have you ever wondered how the chemicals know where to go? How does any curative potion know if you have a headache, an infected finger, or a twisted knee? To begin, you should understand that the MSC cited throughout the literature are really **pericytes** (fibroblasts or cell-signaling proteins) that reside along the exterior lining of blood capillaries. Chief among their functions is to regulate the entry of immune cells into the central nervous system. Physically, the little amoeba-like pericyte works its way along the back of the capillary toward the area of injury, secreting growth factors and looking for sites needing repair. Aspirin, or any other extraneous substance, hitches a ride.

Deep within pericytes are **exosomes**, nanoparticles that conduct the actual signals. Specifically, exosomes are extracellular vesicles generated by all cells, and they carry nucleic acids, proteins, lipids, and metabolites (substances made or used when you metabolize food, chemicals, drugs). Think of them as where all this good stuff is happening. The world of exosomes was largely a theoretical concept until development of high-powered electron microscopes. One scientist who greatly advanced our knowledge of their function was the brilliant cellular biologist Ian White, PhD, who was able to document stem cells in action.

White created a trauma on the tibia of a rat, injected exosomes containing radioactive tracers into the major vein in the rat's tail, and then filmed what took place on the cellular level. The ensuing activity was a real miracle to behold as I could literally see the cells rush to heal. It was yet another epiphany in my quest to discover how to get *un*-glued.

The injected stem cells (pericytes) gathered like a swarm of bees looking for direction. You can see them then react with a form of "intelligence," which speaks to a cellular consciousness that we see throughout the universe. Just like viruses, pericytes are neither good nor evil. They just are. They live to survive. You can see when they sense or recognize a signal from the wound at the rat's leg, heading straight for the injury—straight up the tail, across the torso, and down the leg to the very spot. And as you watch them swarm over the area of trauma and resulting inflammation—the exosomes (filled with **growth factors**—proteins that do the actual repair) get to work. In the world of vascular surgery, shared by Dr. Cooke and others, we call it vascular endothelial growth factor.

A perfect analogy is to think of what it takes to rebuild a house blown apart in a hurricane—you would need all kinds of skills to complete the task: inspectors, architects, construction supervisors, skilled trade workers, and laborers—all working together doing separate tasks geared toward the single goal of rebuilding the house. Now, imagine that your body has suffered damage, not from a hurricane but from sugar, or trauma, or sugar and trauma, causing inflammation, which causes more damage and pain. Like little inspectors on a building project, exosomes enter first, preceding with an axion, the most minute part of a nerve cell.

The exosomes are like cat whiskers probing ahead in the dark, trying to make sense of what they've happened upon. They're looking for the place of injury, communicating with every cell in the damaged area, as if checking its power level. Is this cell okay? Viable enough to survive? Does it need assistance? An energy boost? Or does it need apoptosis—to be killed for the good of the entire organism?

The pericytes in the blood vessels come next, which makes perfect sense. Yet another epiphany for me was that nerves precede vessels in the healing process—well, of course they do. It's like knowing that architects precede contractors. Only, instead of a new building, we have new tissue.

And if you're *rebuilding*, why would you build a network of new tissue into an area of the body that is already dead—or using our house analogy, why would you send builders to a beach site that's already been washed away? You'd build in a place that was solid. So, exosomes scout the location, and pericytes head straight for the worksite where they repair or reproduce tissue as needed. That's healing. That's how the magic happens.

The Stem Cell Crash Course Takeaways

- We all have them. In fact, all human cells originate from stem cells. However, once the developing human is complete, they're concentrated in a few areas and most densely packed in the marrow of our bones.
- In the natural order of things, stem cells are constantly searching for trauma (with its attending inflammation). I hypothesize that the *timing* of stem cell infusions is

related to dosage and, in turn, to results. It's as if giving stem cells soon after acute trauma requires fewer cells and yields faster results. Whereas older chronic trauma with its ensuing fibrosis (scarring from previous inflammation and trauma) takes a higher dose and more time. But, as I've said, that's my working hypothesis.

WHAT'S THE DIFFERENCE?

Everybody knows that medicine has its own vocabulary—generally describing things with words related to how it "presents," what it looks like, and/or how it restricts function. While few people care about medical terminology, to us in the medical field, the difference in definitions is important.

About 30 years ago, I asked Lee Dellon, "Is fibrosis really an "-osis" (an abnormal condition involving an increased number or volume) or is it an "-itis" (meaning inflammation)?"

And he answered, "It's both."

Arthritis is a perfect example. It's red, hot, painful, and swollen—obvious inflammation. Fibrosis is called such because it appears to be a collection of many abnormal cells—a fibrous connective tissue commonly known as a scar.

But fibrosis forms as the result of the body's attempt to heal inflammation—those tiny exosomes trying to rebuild or fill in the damaged space. If you looked at that scar under a microscope, you'd see the striations (ridges or linear markings)—much as your great-grandmother might have darned a sock. If your body's natural fight against sugar must last over time (because you still consume too much sugar), you end up with fibrosis throughout various organs.

And because we've been observing these conditions for eons, we've given them other medical terms such as Alzheimer's, multiple sclerosis, cystitis, etc. In fact, they all are the same thing—different fibrotic reactions at different locations.

- Pulmonary fibrosis or even lung cancer is a great example of the body reacting to chronic irritation and failed attempts at healing. Many scientists even consider some tumors a form of scarring—the body's final efforts at healing a nonhealing wound.

- You can think of a stem cell injection as something akin to chicken soup with bits of healing particles (pericytes, exosomes, and growth factors) suspended in a flavorful sauce. Microbiologists refer to the "sauce" as being packed full of cargo—information being communicated to other cells for the purpose of reconstruction and damage repair. This function is what your own innate stem cells have been doing in your body since your conception. And in our species, for more than 200,000 years.

- Stem cells resolve inflammation and fibrosis. They dissolve the gunk. Think of the process as dissolving the rust of life that has built up, layer upon layer, year after year. That's one reason why stem cell therapy for fibrosis is temporary—the more scar tissue, the harder it is to dissolve. And just as when you're stripping paint off an old

chair or wallpaper in an old house, the more layers you
have, the more solvent you need.[58]

- Animals have them too. Stem cells are species-specific.
  Human stem cells can be grown in laboratories using animal proteins, but these fail in the treatment of humans.
  So far…because scientists are working on genetically
  modifying pig stem cells in hopes that they may successfully cross the species barrier. Cross-species work
  freaks out many people and is at the core of why we—as
  a society—must understand, traverse, and reconcile the
  minefields of science and ethics.

- Your ability to produce optimal stem cells declines with
  age. A cut on a baby's toe can heal in a matter of hours.
  On an octogenarian's toe, it can take weeks or even
  months depending upon the individual's overall health.
  And of course, in many of the cases I see as a peripheral
  nerve surgeon, the cut may not heal at all.

- Stem cells are easy to grow, either from discarded umbilical cord tissue with its wonderous Wharton's jelly[59] or
  from your body's own bone marrow.

- Although only recently examined at the cellular level,
  none of this knowledge is new. When available, ancient
  healers applied placental tissue to battle wounds.

- Current governmental agencies prompted by Big Pharma
  are trying to regulate the cultivation and dissemination
  of therapeutic stem cells just as they currently regulate
  drugs—because that's where the profit is. If you could
  go to a lab and have your own stem cells multiplied and

---

58 More solvent is also needed if you keep repainting the chair or adding more wallpa-
    per (a.k.a., keep eating more sugar).
59 For a more in-depth discussion of Wharton's jelly, see chapter 6.

injected back into you—to heal your cancer, allow you to walk again, stop all pain, *and* extend your lifespan—it would be like saving your own blood for elective surgery (as some people do). Easy peasy and infinitely more economical.

- Some researchers, including Dr. William Li, author of *Eat to Beat Disease*, report that you can *negatively* affect the efficacy of your own stem cells with smoking and inhalation of air pollutants, excessive alcohol consumption, or because of the blood conditions hyperlipidemia (high cholesterol) and hyperglycemia[60] (high glucose). Conversely, you can *positively* affect your stem cells by consuming flavanol-containing cocoa (found in dark chocolate), black tea, and olive oil.

BACK IN PANAMA CITY

We stayed in Panama for a week, and while there I had full access to the facility and many opportunities to speak to the largely Panamanian medical staff—all of whom had been very well trained in modern medicine, primarily at schools in the U.S. However, one physician was from Taiwan, where I used to teach, and we chatted about our mutual experiences in that country. He was a family physician whose ultimate ambition was to obtain a residency in the U.S. I thought to myself, "You want to come to America because you think we have all the medical answers, and yet I'm looking with envy at what you're able to do in your practice and I cannot—because of the political and financial rules of the game."

---

60 In fact, Italian researchers found that that people with diabetes are likely to have 47% *fewer* stem cells as well as stem cells unable to properly function.

I spoke to him about sugar being the cause of all these diseases he was treating with stem cells, and he looked at me in astonishment. "No, that couldn't be the answer; it can't be that simple."

That's the same conversation I'd had in 1981 with Dr. Luke Chu, when he asked me to go to Taiwan to study their emerging epidemic of diabetes and teach in the National Defense Medical School. Dr. Chu, a PhD in pharmacology and surgeon general of the country, was also a four-star general in the Taiwanese army. He was a great golfer and loved the U.S.

Now 40 years later, I was looking at this young doctor, who was mesmerized by modern American medicine. Even though he was also an MD, he couldn't make that connection to the chemical "crème brûlée reaction." The answer is right there—it's sugar, but there's no money in that solution, so people don't look. I hope he figures it out.

RIORDAN'S CLINIC: AUTISM AND STEM CELLS

Most of the patients at Riordan's clinic either had MS or autism (ASD), and it was no surprise. I believe these are the same disease in different nerves. In my opinion, autism involves inflammation mainly of the 12th cranial (hypoglossal[61]) nerve interfacing with the tongue, pharynx, and larynx to affect speech, while MS involves inflammation mainly of the 10th cranial (vagus[62]) nerves. When compressed, they inhibit muscle function throughout the

---

61 The primary nerve to the tongue.
62 Responsible for the parasympathetic systems controlling functions such as heart, breathing, and the immune system.

body. Each of these nerves travel together in very narrow pathways. When inflammation occurs in this constricted space, the result is like what happens in carpal tunnel and tarsal tunnel as discussed in *Sugar Crush* and in part I of this book. And so, after stem cell injections, one of the first symptoms relieved in autism patients is often the inability to speak—and in MS patients, it's the inability to walk steadily unassisted.

One morning I went to the luxurious cafeteria at the clinic where I observed dozens of kids from across the planet, from North America, Asia, Africa, and South America. Beautiful children with facial similarities, regardless of race or age—all with autism.

I've consulted many experts in the autistic world—educators, therapists, physicians, parents. They know the physical appearance of a person on the far end of the autism spectrum. Most will describe the ASD facies—big broad-set eyes and wide upper face, with a decrease in the middle or facial midline. Ears or chins may have been slightly different—but regardless of race or culture, the children resembled one another, as if from the same family. This is because of a single day in gestation when a duplication of a small stretch of protein on the 22nd chromosome leads to a particular facies, or distinctive facial expression, or appearance associated with autism.

Such experts know that those with severe ASD rarely communicate and often seem to be protecting food, eating with their hands and arms in a guarded position. They know they're addicted to sugar! And yet, medical professionals tasked to help individuals with ASD often have no idea of the pathophysiology of a nerve compression. Lack of knowledge of what is going on is the problem.

When I try presenting this theory to my colleagues in the field, they look at me and say, "What are you talking about?" or "What?! How's that possible?"

David Perlmutter, MD, author of bestsellers like *Grain Brain* and *Drop Acid,* affirmed my global compression theory in a June 25, 2022, podcast. He described exactly what's happening, but like the young Taiwanese doc I met at Riordan's clinic, he's not a surgeon, so he didn't make the full connection between sugar and all disease. I'm simply presenting from a different viewpoint. Meanwhile, our patients are being educated into ignorance. We cannot argue that the incidence of autism is increasing in this country, now as high as 1:30 births. It's a disgrace when something as simple as eating sugar is the root cause.

What struck me most that day in the Riordan cafeteria was that the vast majority of parents was feeding their ADS children stacks of muffins and pancakes, orange juice, and other sugar-laden foods. Most striking was that the kids literally hovered over those plates, protecting them as if in fear of someone snatching it away. Of course, I couldn't resist starting a conversation with the woman sitting next to me. She was from Canada but lived in Mexico, and I guessed her son to be about 14 years of age.

Like most of the patients' families, they appeared to be very wealthy, judging by their clothing and jewelry. And you really must be because the therapies can easily cost $20 thousand each, plus transportation and accommodations.[63]

---

63 While a single injury may require only one or two treatments, chronic disease will
    return again and again if sugar remains instrumental in your diet.

I watched the boy eat for a while, shoving in pancakes so fast he could hardly breathe between bites.

"Is this your first time here?" I asked his mother.

"Oh, no," she said. "No, we've been here several times."

"So, do you think this therapy works?"

She replied emphatically, "Absolutely!" She continued, "We spend a week here, and the symptoms go away after he gets his full treatment."

I then asked her, "If it works so well, why do you have to keep coming back?"

"Well, because it doesn't last that long."

"How long does it last?" I asked.

"About a year."

I was fascinated and wanted to know more. She'd brought her son to the clinic several times before, and he had always experienced marked, temporary improvement—sometimes for as long as a year.

"I notice that all these kids seem to love sugar—I wrote a book called Sugar Crush *that you might want to read."*

"Why?" she asked.

"Well, I have this theory it's causing the problem. I think it's a contributing factor in...."

She interrupted, "I don't care—I want my son to have whatever he wants."

The change in her tone was abrupt, but I pressed on. "Well, I notice that he can't speak. Does the therapy allow him to start speaking?"

"Yes," she said. "It's a miracle."

I couldn't resist. "And after that first therapy, when he could speak again, what did he say?"

She thought for a moment and then recalled, "He said, 'I want a donut.'"

I was dumbfounded but managed to reply, "Well, there you go."

With that, she abruptly took her son's hand and led him from the table. By telling her the truth, I'd offended her. And that was the last thing I wanted to do. I'm just the messenger, telling people what I've learned on my own quest to become *un*-glued.

I believe her reaction was in part because Riordan's clinic doesn't stress the causal factors at all. I can understand when patients and doctors think, "What does it matter what causes it, when periodic injections can bring such immediate and profound relief?"

Parents are literally saying, "I have the money; there's a cure. Of course, I'm going to provide for my child the best that money can buy for as long as I can. And if he wants pancakes or donuts, why not?"

It still astonishes me.

WHERE DO THERAPEUTIC STEM CELLS COME FROM?

Allogenic stem cells are transplanted from a donor. **Autologous** stem cells are transplanted from the patient's own body, most often from fat or bone marrow. Each can place a burden not only on selfless, loving donors but particularly on patients. Drilling a hole in someone's bone who's already in a weakened condition after having chemo and/or radiation? Why would you do that? Well, because that's what the law says you must. So as a physician, you're putting a person through an unnecessary procedure— to comply with the current, *misinformed federal law*. That's just sad.

Then there's the matter of shelf life, and 90% of stem cells are dissipated by age 50. Even those lasting over age 50 are weak and puny—far less efficient than are those found in perinatal tissue. (Now that I'm older than most of my patients, I can add, "And because I'm much older than you, my stem cells are named Bernie and George. Those are the only two guys left. So, if I have an "-itis," and it's the middle of the night, Bernie and George don't want to get up and answer the call. They're as tired as I am. 'We don't want to go down where that problem is,' they say. 'Been there, done that.'")

Such a point in our appointment is when I tell an older patient that it would be disingenuous for me to proceed with autologous therapy—to take your money and put you through an invasive and unnecessary procedure, when there is another, simpler third alternative. I explain that you will prosper more with an IV of young, fully invigorated clones from amniotic fluid and umbilical cord that would ordinarily be labeled medical waste and discarded. Dr. Riordan doesn't use bone marrow aspirant in Panama; he uses allogenic perinatal tissue—umbilical tissue, Wharton's jelly—just as I do. Are they stem cells or not?

No doubt the preferred nomenclature regarding stem cells can quickly turn esoteric. For instance, I've completed the online course presented by the Perinatal Stem Cell Society, with lectures from the leaders in the field: Joanne Kurtzberg, Ian White, and Arnold Caplan (who named them MSC)—and they all have differing viewpoints on the correct name.[64]

But the whole circular discussion can be boiled down to this: in utero, as the fetus is developing, amnionic tissue bathes it in amnionic fluid where there is a constant exchange of stem cells from the placenta to the umbilical cord to the fluid itself, and back—all in service of building a human being. But as soon as a child is ready to be born, the mother's body expels the fluid, as it's no longer needed. Once the umbilical cord is cut upon the baby's delivery, it's no longer needed, with the same result when the mother naturally expels the placenta—that is, it's discarded. Tissue coming from these three sources *are* still filled with functioning stem cells, but after processing (which can include preservatives, freezing, unfreezing, and counting), they do not have an in vitro recipient. Thus, they are "not living," so you can't really call them "stem cells."

It may seem like hair-splitting semantics, but that's how science operates. And that's why it's important to call them what they really are: pericytes and growth factors. They're still miraculous when you think about how, even then, they can still trigger another body to repair, rebuild, and rejuvenate. So, I applaud you

---

64 Not the least of which is why Caplan named them mesenchymal stem cells when they're really pericytes, a decision he's since walked back.

who become pregnant. You literally hold the survival of the species. You are the guardians of life—the true *células madre*.

AHEAD OF THE CURVE

In Panama, Jim received cells taken from the Wharton's jelly of the umbilical cord. Once retrieved, they were *grown or cultured* in a broth (expanding the tissue volume) and finally given intravenously—going from the laboratory to the IV in his arm in a day or two.

We are prohibited from cultivating human cells in the U.S. The reasons why, along with the vagaries of U.S. law (primarily written by Big Pharma), will be explored in a later chapter.

None of the U.S. regulations currently in place address whether or not the treatment works. The answer is yes—it works on anything. I can assure you of that truth in person during our consult. I can't advertise it because I haven't done the research on every single "-itis" or "osis" for which it will be used (as demanded by the FDA). And how many of those are there? Is it 15,000?

Doing the research for each illness costs millions, in part because it must be done over 10 years. Who has the capability of doing that? Big Pharma, which farms it out to large, wealthy medical schools. And yet, how much research do you need to do before you realize that without *any* therapy, the patient is going to die? I feel this issue is a moral and ethical question—particularly for dying patients, where all else has failed already. Why not allow the treatment?

I recently read of an infant with an extremely rare genetic disease involving the gap gene found in the mammalian glycocalyx—that glorious layer consisting of glucose, proteins, and lipids that surrounds and protects each human cell. In such instances, an appropriate sugar can develop, but it can't attach properly to all the other tissues, so these kids have severe, life-threatening symptoms.

Her name is Lucy, and she probably will not live to her first birthday. Meanwhile, she has severe autistic-like symptoms: she cannot speak; she cannot move; she cannot swallow; she cannot thrive.

All these brilliant scientists are working on it, writing the paper describing it. And I say to myself, "Why don't they try *stem cells!*" I just think so differently. I want to scream to the world: "Why would you even debate this? The child is going to die otherwise. What have you got to lose? You're too smart; you're trying to overthink it. Just give it to her. Anything else is cruel."

If I were the parent of a child dying from this anomaly of the gap gene, or from an aggressive brain tumor known as a glioblastoma, and I learned—not from my doctor but another source—that stem cell therapy could make a difference, I wouldn't hesitate. And yet, I believe that knowledge is being kept from us, in part, because it will do away with most modern medical practices.

HOW THE U.S. FELL BEHIND IN STEM CELL RESEARCH

Time for a quick brain-break review. As discussed earlier, there are four main categories of stem cells:

- Embryonic—premature cells in the earliest stages of pre-birth development.

- Adult—a catch-all phrase for stems cells existing after birth.

- Altered adult—cells taken from a living person or cadaver, then reprogrammed to react more like embryonic stem cells.

- Perinatal—cells that bathe and nurture the fetus. They're contained in amnionic fluid, umbilical cord tissue, and placental tissue.

Because there are so many renditions of the stem cell song, intermixed with moral, social, semantic, and intimately personal philosophies, we can't all sing the same tune.

In 2004, the U.S. Senate held seminal hearings, chaired by Senator John McCain, in which celebrated expert witnesses all proclaimed that stem cell therapy not only worked, but that it could radically change American medicine! Many including former Senator Sam Brownback, from the great state of Kansas and now a fellow with the Center for Religious Liberty, even used the word "miracle." Yet, the bioethics were left unresolved, and President George W. Bush reinforced his 2001 ban on funding for clinical research using human embryonic stem cells.

Currently in the U.S., researchers can still get embryonic stem cell clonal lines that were established before the ban instituted by Bush, but they cannot establish new ones. So, for the past 20 years, the medical field has inched forward. At one point, the Mayo Clinic mission statement declared that they would not be doing *medicine* in the future but rather working with stem cells. There was even talk of building a stem cell "factory" in Jacksonville, Florida. That proposal has since been walked back.

A sidebar to the Senate hearing was that the prescription drug plan under Medicare was happening around that time—and Big Pharma was trying to kill it. The idea of adding inexpensive stem cells for all to the bill was a bridge too far for that industry. Legislators aren't always adept at discussing and compromising on the moral/ethical issues inherent in any scientific progress. Specifically in the case of stem cells, opposition came in the specter of human cloning—and an age-old fear that, once freed from the underworld, some mad Frankenstein would cobble together an interspecies abomination.

Now, 20 years later, Big Pharma and large medical conglomerates are obstructing progress on *any* stem cell research so that they can maintain control of the *trillion-dollar* drug monopoly. In the meantime, the real question should be "Why does society need pain killers when stem cells can repair fibrosis and regenerate tissue?" Stop the pain caused by the oft-maligned "too-simple-to-be-true cause." Yes, and remember you heard it here—sugar. The next chapter, "Why You Can't Get Them at Walgreens," explores those successful stall tactics.

Bibliography

Caplan, Arnold I. "Mesenchymal Cells: Time to Change the Name!" *Stem Cells Translational Medicine* 6, no. 6 (2017): 1445–1521. https://doi.org/10.1002/sctm.17-0051.

Chatterjee, Rangan. "The Key Driver of Chronic Disease That Nobody's Talking About with David Perlmutter." June 7, 2023. In *Feel Better, Live More*. Podcast. MP3 audio. 1:17:37. https://drchatterjee.com/the-key-driver-of-chronic-disease-that-nobodys-talking-about-with-david-perlmutter/.

Adult Stem Cell Research: Successes from the Field: Hearing on S. HRG 108-959, Before the Subcommittee on Science, Technology, and Space of the Committee on Commerce, Science, and Transportation. 108th Congress, Second Session. July 14, 2004. https://www.govinfo.gov/content/pkg/CHRG-108shrg81637/pdf/CHRG-108shrg81637.pdf.

Fadini, Gian Paolo, Marta Miorin, Monica Facco, Sondra Bonamico, Ilenia Baesso, Franco Grego, Mirko Menegolo, Saula Vigili de Kreutzenberg, Antonio Tiengo, Carlo Agostini, and Angelo Avogaro. "Circulating Endothelial Progenitor Cells Are Reduced in Peripheral Vascular Complications of Type 2 Diabetes Mellitus." *Journal of the American College of Cardiology* 45, no. 9 (2005): 1449–1457. https://doi.org/10.1016/j.jacc.2004.11.067.

Forrest, Richard D. "Early History of Wound Treatment." *Journal of the Royal Society of Medicine* 75, no. 3 (1982): 198–205. https://doi.org/10.1177/014107688207500310.

Frontiers Editorial Office. "Retraction: Deep Learning for Autism Diagnosis and Facial Analysis in Children." *Frontiers*

in Computational Neuroscience 17 (2023): https://doi.
    org/10.3389/fncom.2023.1215827.

Grassi, Davide, Richard Draijer, Casper Schalkwij,
    Giovambattista Desideri, Anatolia D'Angeli, Sandro
    Francavilla, Theo Mulder, and Claudio Ferri. "Black
    Tea Increases Circulating Endothelial Progenitor Cells
    and Improves Flow Mediated Dilatation Counteracting
    Deleterious Effects from a Fat Load in Hypertensive
    Patients: A Randomized Controlled Study." *Nutrients* 8, no.
    11 (2016): 727–758. https://doi.org/10.3390/nu8110727.

Heiss, Christian, Sarah Jahn, Melanie Taylor, Wendy May Real,
    Franca S. Angeli, Maelene L. Wong, Nicolas Amabile,
    Megha Prasad, Tienush Rassaf, Javier I. Ottaviani, Shirley
    Mihardja, Carl L. Keen, Matthew L. Springer, Andrew
    Boyle, William Grossman, Stanton A. Glantz, Hagen
    Schroeter, and Yerem Yeghiazarians. "Improvement of
    Endothelial Function with Dietary Flavanols Is Associated
    with Mobilization of Circulating Angiogenic Cells in
    Patients with Coronary Artery Disease." *Journal of the
    American College of Cardiology* 56, no. 3 (2010): 218–224.
    https://doi.org/10.1016/j.jacc.2010.03.039.

Hosseini, Mohammad-Parsa, Madison Beary, Alex Hadsell, Ryan
    Messersmith, and Hamid Soltanian-Zadeh. "RETRACTED:
    Deep Learning for Autism Diagnosis and Facial Analysis
    in Children." *Frontiers in Computational Neuroscience* 15
    (2021): https://doi.org/10.3389/fncom.2021.789998.

Karacaer, Cengiz, Selcuk Yaylaci, Taner Demirci, Deniz Cekic,
    Kezban Ozmen Suner, Erdem Cokluk, and Ceyhun Varim.
    "Association of Mortality and Endothelial Dysfunction
    with Serum ADMA Level in COVID-19 Patients." *Pakistan*

Journal of Medical Science 38, no. 7 (2022): 1808–1815. https://doi.org/10.12669/pjms.38.7.5327.

Li, William W. *Eat to Beat Disease: The New Science of How Your Body Can Heal Itself.* London: Balance Books, 2021.

Marin, Carmen, Rafael Ramirez, Javier Delgado-Lista, Elena Maria Yubero-Serrano, Pablo Perez-Martinez, Julia Carracedo, Antonio Garcia-Rios, Fernando Rodriguez, Francisco Miguel Gutierrez-Mariscal, Purificación Gomez, Francisco Perez-Jimenez, and José López-Miranda. "Mediterranean Diet Reduces Endothelial Damage and Improves the Regenerative Capacity of Endothelium." *The American Journal of Clinical Nutrition* 93, no. 2 (February 2011): 267–274. https://doi.org/10.3945/ajcn.110.006866.

Rodier, Patricia M. "The Early Origins of Autism." *Scientific American* 282, no. 2 (2000): 56–63. https://doi.org/10.1038/scientificamerican0200-56.

"Stem Cell Institute." Riordan Technologies. Accessed April 16, 2024. https://www.neilriordan.com/stem-cell-institute/.

Tripi, Gabriele, Sylvie Roux, Domenica Matranga, Laura Maniscalco, Pasqualino Glorioso, Frédérique Bonnet-Brilhault, and Michele Roccella. "Cranio-Facial Characteristics in Children with Autism Spectrum Disorders (ASD)." *Journal of Clinical Medicine* 8, no. 5 (2019): 641. https://doi.org/10.3390/jcm8050641.

CHAPTER 6

Why You Can't Get
Them at Walgreens

—governance and greed

In 1981, scientists first learned how to extract stem cells from mouse embryos early in their development. Just 17 years later, biologist James Alexander Thomson devised a means of extracting stem cells from *human embryos* (unused and donated from in vitro fertilization) and growing those cells in the laboratory. With this momentous step came recognition of their remarkable regenerative potential and the promise of life-saving cures and therapies for humanity.

Then, on August 9, 2001, in part because of his personal ethical considerations, President George W. Bush introduced a ban on federal funding of research on newly created human embryonic stem (ES) cell lines[65] and thus strengthened the Dickey-Wicker amendment, a law passed by Congress in 1996 that prohibits

---

65 Remember these cells are pluripotent, meaning they can develop into any type of cell. They're also sometimes called perinatal or birth tissue.

"federally funded investigators from creating or causing harm to embryos."

By way of compromise, researchers were still allowed to maintain, reproduce, and use cells from the ES cell lines then in existence, but as you can imagine, those resources are finite and declining. The action spurred a debate firestorm regarding the ethical and moral definitions of life—prompting many scientists (including Neil Riordan) to leave this country in search of other sources of ES cells for both research and regenerative therapy.[66]

Patients often say, "I don't want stem cells; it seems like you're harming a baby somehow." While understandable, such concern is simply unwarranted. It's been said earlier, but it bears repeating: The *therapeutic* use of human ES cells remains illegal throughout the U.S. And you don't need human ES cells for healing when nonembryonic adult stem cells provide the same healing benefits.

However, it's important here to distinguish between federal and state regulations regarding the use of human ES cells *for research*—and the use of **non**-ES cells for *either research or therapeutic* purposes.

In reaction to Bush's federal ban on human ES research, and one year after the McCain Senate hearings of 2003, the voters of California passed the California Research and Cures Initiative. In this amendment, the state constitution made stem cell research a constitutional right. This action led to creation of the California

---

66 Riordan is now using nonembryonic stems cells derived from Wharton's jelly found in the umbilical cord.

Institute for Regenerative Medicine—an institution to fund, facilitate, and provide oversight for stem cell research in that state. In 2009, President Barack Obama signed an executive order overturning Bush's original federal ban on using human ES cells in research. In the intervening years, 29 states have stepped in with laws restricting use of human ES cells for research, while 11 have enacted total bans. Calling it a volatile and complicated landscape is an understatement.

THE BEAT GOES ON

In a separate venue under the Public Health Services Act, the FDA is empowered to regulate human cells, tissue, and secretions used for *therapeutic* purposes—and it does so by designating them as either a **Section 351** "product" or a **Section 361** "product."[67] The regulations officially refer to this material as "human cells, tissues, and cellular and tissue-based products" or "HCT/Ps"—but for simplicity's sake, I'll use the generic term "stem cells" going forward.

The FDA considers any Section 351 product to be a *drug*, and thus it must undergo extensive clinical trials. Not only are the trials required for every iteration of every product as it relates to every iteration of every disease, but they also take years and millions of dollars to complete. Those requirements are why the gateway to the development of stem cell therapies only exists via partnerships between Big Pharma (the money) and medical universities and institutions (folks with a steady supply of time, trained personnel, and scientific expertise). If a single physician

---

67 The labels are based on the specific sections of the regulatory statute.

wants to conduct a clinical trial, it must be privately financed or politically correct (meaning nonthreatening financially or politically to the gatekeepers). However, physicians and other licensed health care providers may self-regulate their use of products deemed to fall into Section 361. As with most federal regulations, they're purposefully byzantine—but to fully appreciate the health benefits we're being denied, I believe it's imperative to recognize the lengths to which legislators, at the behest of Big Pharma, have cloaked the topic. So, let's give it a go.

A Crash Course on Federal Standards for the Therapeutic Use of Human Stem Cells[68]

Rule #1: Following the same restrictions placed on all drugs, a health care provider cannot administer, dispense, or prescribe stem cells not first approved for human use by the U.S. Food and Drug Administration. An FDA stamp of approval pretty much defines a **Section 351** product.

Rule #2: A health care provider must maintain medical records on each patient.

Rule #3: Those records must include documentation of diagnosis and purpose of use.

Rule #4: There are exceptions to the FDA regulations.

Don't be fooled by this early flight of simplicity because the exceptions are where they've planted the hedges that comprise the maze.

---

68 Distilled from the actual federal regulations so you don't have to.

The Exceptions to Rule #4:

a. The health care provider has been approved for an Investigational New Drug application—the first step in the long road to Section 351 approval. The next steps involve the years and moneys required to establish a specific clinical trial. The last step before approval is the Institutional Review Board.

b. The health care provider is operating in a federally approved trial certified by the Foundation of Accreditation of Cellular Therapy, the NIH clinical trials network/ Blood and Marrow Transplant Clinical Trials Network, or the American Association of Blood Banks. These are primarily grandfathered research facilities funded by Big Pharma, the federal government, and associated foundations.

c. Autologous use. The health care provider is removing stem cells from one individual and implanting them in the same individual. So, just as you can harvest your own blood before elective surgery, a physician may take blood marrow stem cells from your own pelvic bone and inject it into another injured or diseased blood-related part of your own body.[69] The problem is that the number and potency of your stem cells begins to decline at about age 20, and they're 90% gone after age 50.

---

69 Typical uses are for blood cancers such as leukemia, multiple myeloma, and non-Hodgkin's lymphoma, as well as for blood diseases such as sickle cell anemia.

d. The health care provider self-regulates the stem cell "product" according to the conditions outlined in regulation 21 CFR 1271.10. Now, we're at the controversial heart of **Section 361**. These are the conditions:

- Stem cells must be minimally manipulated (no freaky cloning or interspecies stuff).

- Therapy is for homologous use only. The word is of Greek origins and means "like for like"—either on the structural or cellular level. It means that transplanted cells must fulfill the same use or function in the recipient's body as they did in the donor's body. Your health care provider may take blood marrow stem cells (yours or another's) and use them to treat your blood disease (most often cancer). Your health care provider may *not* take stem cells from, say, a heart valve and use them to treat brain cancer.

- When "processing" stem cells they may not be combined with any other article except water, crystalloids,[70] or preservatives.

- The stem cell product must meet one of these requirements:

    i. It must not have a systemic effect (affect the whole body) or be dependent upon the metabolic activity of living cells.

OR

---

70 Intravenous electrolyte solutions used in hospitals and emergency interventions to stabilize bodily fluids.

ii. If it *does* have a systemic effect or *is* dependent upon the metabolic activity of living cells it must meet these criteria:

- Be tissue from the same person (autologous use).
- Be tissue from another person (allogeneic use) who is a first-degree or second-degree blood relative.[71]
- Be used for reproduction.

e. Other uses approved by the FDA (just in case they should want to).

As these regulations sink in, ponder the following health care scenario. "Live" cells, secretions, or tissue having metabolic activity are officially labeled as "drugs" and thus require the more complex Section 351 designation. Amnionic fluid is a secretion, meaning that it's considered to be a drug. I find that incredible. Without FDA authorization, a woman may not use her own amnionic fluid to ease the suffering of a dying spouse—or a blood-related adopted child—or anyone else with whom she has an abiding philosophical/moral/spiritual human connection. To obtain authorization, a health care provider facilitating such an exchange must file for a new drug application through a legitimate Institutional Review Board. That process will cost millions of dollars and will take five to 10 years to complete. Moreover, to receive FDA 351 approval, this "product" must have undergone clinical trials designed for each specific use. The constraint includes every iteration of a cell, tissue, or secretion and every

---

71 A first-degree blood relative is a parent, sibling, or child. A second-degree blood relative is when there is only one other genetic relative between you and the donor—such as grandparent and grandchild, half siblings, aunt/uncle and niece/nephew.

iteration of every disease—all to prove what we already know is safe and effective for use on anything.

WHAT IS THIS FDA ACRONYM ANYWAY?

When the FDA was established in the early 1900s, it was designed to protect the American public from quacks, hucksters, snake-oil salesmen, barrow boys, and assorted carnival acts. And it was to be funded with tax dollars appropriated by Congress and approved by the president—a noble cause in service of the public interest. And yet…

It is *no accident* that today 75% of the FDA's $1.1 billion drug-division budget comes from the pharmaceutical industry it was created to regulate. These moneys are part of the user fees paid by companies seeking FDA approval for drugs and devices. Such fees—as well as "performance measures," which include the time it takes to approve or reject a new drug or product—are negotiated in closed-door meetings among Big Pharma lobbyists, Congress, and White House officials.[72] In fact, as reported by *The New York Times* and others, the FDA doesn't even attend the negotiations.

Put yourself in Big Pharma's shoes for a minute. If you profited from a *trillion*-dollar drug industry that covers up pain rather than curing the cause of it, would *you* gleefully encourage stem cell therapies that would put you out of the drug business? Or would you encourage and fund complex regulatory systems? Control research and patents? Keep medical schools and institutions flush

---

72 Outside the meetings, lobbyists reported spending an *additional* $373.74 million in 2022 to wine, dine, and further "educate" their fellow committee members regarding the ROI of R&D (a.k.a., why drug prices *must* cost so much).

with endowment moneys? I've said it before (and will to my dying breath), Big Pharma makes all deals when it comes to health care.

HOW DO THESE REGULATIONS AFFECT THE PATIENTS I SEE DAILY?

A woman came to my clinic 15 years ago with advanced and very painful Achilles tendonitis. She was a nurse and fully understood the extent of the damage—she'd also been to several physicians before me.

After patiently answering my questions regarding her medical history, she quickly asked if I could use platelet-rich plasma (PRP) injections to alleviate her constant pain. A precursor to current regenerative methods, PRP is an autologous treatment in which the patient's own blood is drawn, then processed to extract growth factors that when reinjected will initiate healing.

I asked how long she'd been experiencing the pain.

"A year and a half."

"I see you're wearing a cast boot," I said. *"How long have you been wearing that?"*

And again, she answered, "A year and a half."

"Why do you want PRP?"

"Because I had it done on my elbow, and it worked there. I'm not taking any more opioids. I don't see why in the world you couldn't use it on my heel."

Clearly, I wasn't the first to have heard this plea. As matter of fact, I had used PRP therapies. Serendipitously, at her appointment with me, a company producing a new stem cell product (at that time touted as a form of "amnionic fluid") was visiting the clinic, so I asked if she'd like to sit in on their presentation to our staff.

"Listen to what they have to say, and let's evaluate it together."

Later, she eagerly opted for the amniotic treatment, and the day after her first injection, my examination revealed no inflammation—zero pain or tenderness. We both were astonished that it had happened so quickly. I suggested she keep the boot on for another two weeks, to be extra cautious. But when she returned, there was still no inflammation, no pain. Now, 15 years later, she has not had a recurrence.

I know now that what the manufacturer was then calling amnionic stem cells was actually a reduction of growth factors and cytokines[73]—not something as simple as pure amnionic fluid. Nevertheless, it has since been deemed an unapproved Section 351 product, which means that without exhaustive and expensive clinical trials, it can only be used legally if your physician goes through the Investigational New Drug application, then through an Institutional Review Board—for *each* patient and *each* instance. Just more hoops to jump through until official FDA approval.

The reasoning behind such restrictions always goes like this: "Well, we want to be *super safe*, so we need a huge amount of overlapping research. We're only looking out for the well-being of the patient."

---

73 Microscopic proteins secreted in the immune system and used for cell signaling.

With that in mind, I came upon a recent blog by Dr. Todd Peters, a board-certified orthopedic and spine surgeon in Newport Beach, California. In it he writes: "Stem cell therapy is more advanced than PRP therapy... [it] not only does the same thing that PRP offers, which is initiating the body's repair response, it also enhances stem cell activity for regeneration."

And yet, if my same patient were to walk into my office again today with Achilles tendonitis, I would be unable to administer the same treatment I used 15 years ago. She'd be flat out of luck because to my knowledge, no researcher has yet conducted a trial for the specific application of this specific formula to the specific condition of Achilles tendonitis.

It's a perfect example of how the pharmaceutical regulatory apparatus has slow-walked a treatment known to be safe and effective. I'm convinced the industry applies its pressure so that stem cell therapy can be controlled by Big Pharma. After all, who needs expensive drugs if you can simply use stem cells for all injury and disease?

That conundrum leaves us with the few options we can exercise.

WHARTON'S JELLY: A SECTION 351 OR 361 PRODUCT?

Earlier, I mentioned Wharton's jelly as the rich, gelatinous substance within and surrounding the umbilical cord and placenta. It's considered an "adult" perinatal substance and used by health care providers across the country, including myself. I've seen it work miracles—not only in my patients but as mentioned in chapter 5 when treating my own herniated disc shoulder pain and ripped plantaris tendon.

Nevertheless, Wharton's jelly continues to be the subject of professional friction between the FDA and those of us practicing in regenerative therapies. FDA regulators have been persistent in challenging individuals using Wharton's jelly, as well as companies manufacturing it, contending that, like amnionic fluid, it, too, is a drug, thus falling within their auspices and Section 351 of the Public Health Services Act. However, many scientists, manufacturers, and practitioners challenge that presumption. Our position is that precisely *because* it's a naturally occurring substance, Wharton's jelly is not a "drug." When it's been minimally manipulated and used for homologous use, it clearly meets Section 361 criteria.

Many leaders in the regenerative field concede that under the FDA criteria of "homologous," it's a stretch to say that Wharton's jelly could be injected into, say, a patient's damaged knee joint. Given the current FDA parameters, I would agree. However, I wouldn't agree that the treatment doesn't work—because it does. To go around this technical roadblock, others in the industry maintain that Wharton's jelly has a "cushioning effect" in a damaged knee— making it feel better. That's also true. It does. Its application *still* doesn't neatly fit into the FDA definition of homologous use. I strongly believe the disparity is because the FDA definition is incomplete—it simply doesn't go far enough.

The logical extension of the definition is actually quite apparent. In the purest sense, a fetus is like any other end organ in the mother's body—her heart, liver, etc. The umbilical cord, of course, is the physical connection between fetus and mother. Even knowing full well of its cultural volatility, I use the word "fetus" because it's the medical term before the moment of birth—before the cord is cut. At this time of attachment, healing cells within the cord are called embryonic stem cells.

The umbilical cord contains one vein delivering nutrients to the fetus and two arteries removing waste and taking it back to the placenta for processing and eventual elimination.[74] This conduit thus services every eye, muscle, and joint of the developing human being.

Wharton's jelly is the protective sheath cushioning and protecting the cord—or conduit—of life. I emphasize the word "conduit" because it is one of the words used in the FDA's definition of a structural or homologous usage. And as the fetus develops— still bathed in stem cells—and forms its own conduits to its own organs, it begins to supply nutrients to every organ system and, conversely, removes waste. In this regard, every stem cell within a sample of umbilical cord is homologous to *every* part of the human body—supplying every end organ of a human being.

Then the cord is cut.

After the cut, cells from the discarded umbilical cord with its Wharton's jelly (still bathed in and filled with the exosomes and growth factors) are called adult stem cells.

---

74 This is unique in the umbilical cord as arteries usually carry nutrients, while veins carry waste. There's also an immature nerve structure that (while it lacks the nerve endings necessary to carry a pain sensation to either mother or fetus)—does have a cholinergic (or chemical) effect that transmits information.

In the postnatal body, conduits functioning like the umbilical cord are called neurovascular bundles—structures comprised of veins, arteries, and nerves that all travel in tandem to specific tissue. While mainstream orthodoxy does not yet recognize that these bundles exist in every end organ (making them universal throughout the body), Dellon made the homologous connection between the arm and leg, proving the double-crush syndrome of Upton and McComas. The universality of the concept seems obvious to me.

A simple analogy is the way in which electricity moves through a building. Somewhere outside of the building is a transformer that directs electricity to the structure and in turn to all the wires leading to outlets and eventually to end terminals known as lamps, appliances, air conditioners, etc. Supportive function meets that definition for a conduit—exactly as my global compression theory postulates.

After birth, we all retain innate living stem cells allowing us to continue growing until about age 20 when they begin to decline. And as discussed earlier, by age 50 and thereafter, living stem cells are 90% gone. As a physician, I ask myself, wouldn't returning umbilical tissue (especially Wharton's jelly) to someone 70 or 80 years of age and replete of their own stem cells be returning *like to like*? Conduit to conduit?

When viewed through this lens, the function of Wharton's jelly *is* homologous and thus Section 361 compliant. More specifically, the definition of the action of Wharton's jelly to prevent compression is the sine qua non of the homologous use in the FDA's Section 361 guidelines. If the global compression theory doesn't fit that definition, then federal regulators have made a category that is unobtainable. Unconscionable!

In my surgical practice, I apply Wharton's jelly around the neurovascular bundles in the legs and feet—and the results are a relief of pain, quickly followed by a full regenerative process. It's also important to note that Wharton's jelly technically does not contain *living* stem cells once it's out of the natal environment.

As science moves forward, the legal battles lumber to catch up. Late in 2022, amid all the scientific discussions and dozens of court cases, the FDA sued the California Stem Cell Treatment Center, charging that stem cells in general are drugs requiring FDA approval before they could be sold. In a seminal decision, the court ruled that stem cells *are not* a drug but rather a naturally occurring substance, fundamentally blocking the FDA's ability to regulate stem cell therapies at all.

Of course, the FDA has filed an appeal to the U.S. Court of Appeals for the 9th Circuit. Meanwhile, this lower court decision is at odds with decisions handed down in other states regarding similar or the same regenerative products. No doubt all claims will eventually end up in the Supreme Court, so stay tuned by visiting https://www.drjacoby.academy/courses/unglued.

SMALL-FIBER VS. LARGE-FIBER PERIPHERAL NEUROPATHY

Most of my patients come to me and other podiatrists because they're experiencing the tingling, burning pain, and uncontrollable itching of the legs or feet—small-fiber peripheral neuropathy.

It's commonly experienced by people who copresent with diabetes. Meanwhile, those with large-fiber neuropathy (loss of muscle function) generally are referred to a neurologist.

Large-fiber neuropathy presents as loss of muscle function in the extremities (hands, feet, arms, legs) as well as symptoms including weakness, a vibrating sensation, and loss of balance or coordination.[75] Throughout my training and early practice, scientists thought these were two separate diseases.

Then in 2004, I was asked to give a presentation at the Smithsonian Institution on the distinction of the two types of neuropathy. After some research, I was hard-pressed to clearly see, let alone define, a distinction. It didn't make sense to me. I consulted with my mentor Lee Dellon and Sonny Yamasaki, a PhD neuroanatomist who is currently the director of new therapy development at Medtronic in Minnesota. They both insisted that the two diseases were separate. I still wasn't getting it.

I smile when I remember how these two renowned scientists quoted all the relevant Nobel laureates and patiently repeated, "You don't understand."

I replied, "I understand what you're saying—I don't agree." I was convinced I was right, but who was I to say so?

Then, with the speech still looming overhead, my family and I left for a long-anticipated vacation in Great Britain where I found myself sitting in the Eurostar terminal, waiting to board the

---

75 Neurologists often use the term "dysautonomia" to describe the bundle of these same symptoms.

train that travels 100 mph through the tunnel under the English Channel, connecting England and France. We'd just visited the Queen Square hospital, where Dr. Henry Schutta, a neurologist and one of my old professors, had trained. He was a fascinating guy who told great stories and practiced until he was 92 years old. Dr. Schutta always insisted we use the Queen Square reflex hammer—a long instrument allowing us to reach over the beds at Pennsylvania Hospital to tap and test the large muscle fiber response in neurology patients.[76] I thoroughly enjoyed the memories. Still, I'd promised my wife a trip to Paris and the kids a ride through the "chunnel" as a reward for the little side trip.

As we sat waiting for the train to Paris, the speech weighed heavily on my mind because I didn't really know what I was going to say. I still wasn't clear on the topic of small-fiber versus large-fiber neuropathies, but I had to get up in front of this huge group—at the Smithsonian of all places!

Frustrated, I looked around the terminal, which is like a gigantic, covered semicircular amphitheater with the tracks seeming to come from the audience to converge center stage—and on into the tunnel. Instinctively I thought, "Oh, that looks like a neurovascular interchange where the axions transfer energy to the nerves." At the same time, I heard the surrounding hordes speaking dozens of languages—which was like all the different proteins trying to communicate with one another. I had the opening for my speech!

You need to be on a train in a tunnel or subway to get this experience, but suddenly, it all made sense. Imagine that the Eurostar

---

76 I know, I know, but a trip to an old professor's alma mater is exactly the kind of vacation excursion I'm apt to take.

is like a nerve going into a bone tunnel. Moving from small- to large-fiber neuropathy is like coming to a stop at the end of that ride—and it's a four-phase process.

Approaching the station in France, there was the screeching of brakes on wheels with sparks coming off—the earliest phase of friction for the train, like the axion hitting the nerve wall as inflammation causes it to constrict. You might feel the train gently rocking to and fro, but it's no big deal. That's phase one. Suddenly, the screeching gets louder as the train brakes more—that's phase two. Phase three would be if you were going to crash. The train's wheels would lock up. You'd be jerked forward, and there'd be a different, more horrible sound and the smell of smoke. At phase four, all would probably go quiet until phase five—when you'd come to a full stop. You're going nowhere. You're stuck in the tunnel.

Don't be surprised, but 20 years later, I've been proven correct about small-fiber versus large-fiber neuropathies. We now know (because of ADMA and the work I did with John Cooke) that both exist along a continuum. They are phases in the same process. The process starts as a chemical reaction to sugar and involves the tiny unmyelinated C-fiber nerves,[77] which are responsible for the transfer of sensations such as temperature, pain, and itching. As the disease progresses, the diameter of those fibers gets bigger—there's a layered buildup of myeline, more insulation, less energy going through the nerve into the A and B motor fibers that move muscles.

---

77 These nerves are unmyelinated, meaning they are not covered with a thin protective coating. Nerves with myeline coverings are called A and B fiber depending upon the amount of coating.

Can there be a genetic "doesn't-matter-what-the-hell-you-eat" factor to large-fiber neuropathy? Yes, such a disease has been identified as purely genetic, and it's a rare condition called Tangier disease. But in most cases, large-fiber neuropathy is a simple progression that's caused by sugar. And because of the increasing volume of processed foods in the typical diet, we are now seeing a huge increase in the numbers of patients with both large- and small-fiber neuropathies.

Statistics on small-fiber neuropathy are rare (primarily because for years patients can ignore intermittent symptoms—primarily pain—or mask them with OTC pain killers). Data published by NIH cites that 10 million to 20 million Americans over the age of 40 seek professional relief for the condition—accounting for over $10 billion in health care costs per year. A study conducted by scientists with the Mayo Clinic followed patients over a six-year period with incidence rising from 1.3 per 100,000 per year to 13.3.

It can take up to 40 years for small-fiber neuropathy to progress into large-fiber neuropathy and severe muscle impairment—so we have yet to see the full tsunami awaiting us. The tsunami includes all those individuals currently being told they have prediabetes, metabolic syndrome, fibromyalgia, polymyalgia, impaired glucose tolerance, and all the other buzzwords we physicians can use for conditions not fully understood. As with other conditions such as shingles and anxiety, Lyrica works great to relieve the symptoms by blocking pain transmission in the brain. However, without removing sugar from one's diet, the underlying cause will simply progress. Lyrica does not solve the problem—it merely monetizes it.

STEM CELLS AND NEUROPATHIES

In years past, upon first examination, three out of 100 of my patients would have immediately needed surgery. The rest could have been treated with drugs such as Lyrica that didn't get to the root of the cause but could at least relieve the painful symptoms. Then, I became fully aware of the regenerative properties of stem cells, and I slowly began giving the same conservative dosage to everyone. Soon, I recognized that they could work even in my older patients—chipping away at the long-term scarring that had been building up for decades.

If you come to me with small-fiber neuropathy today—the first phase in a sugar-driven continuum—I would not use stem cell therapy. I'd counsel you to change your diet, as if putting oil on the squeaky wheels, and the symptoms would probably go away.

If you progress into phase two, you've still got a chance and wouldn't need stem cells, but we'd know that you needed to try harder with the diet. Look more closely for the hidden sugars.

But at phase three, your brakes are locked, and you're heading for a crash. This phase is the perfect place to initiate stem cells because they will immediately reduce the inflammation and begin regeneration.

At phase four, when I tap on the nerve with my Queen Square hammer, you have no reflexes. You now have large-fiber neuropathy, and your muscles are being affected.

Phase five is when you hit stop.

Dellon would say that at this point, if you have a negative Hoffman-Tenel sign (meaning tapping on the nerve and nothing happens)—amputation is the only course of action. It's as if you must be extracted from that train car. You're stuck—you must get out or you're dead.

I have used stem cells in phase five, and sensation *can* return because those nerves may not really be dead—they may not be transmitting signals. So, we don't give up. However, when the nerves get necrotic, with actual decay of surrounding tissue, you can't change that. Amputation is the only answer. Obviously we want to catch you before that happens—which is why I've written this book.

MONOCLONAL ANTIBODIES

Since COVID, I'll often have a patient who asks about mono-clonal antibodies for relief of arthritis pain. These are synthetic antibodies that in some cases can act almost as an interim or bridge until the full availability of *affordable* stem cells.

Currently, there are at least a hundred of these drugs for every "-itis" you can think of—the most well-known of which (because of celebrity endorsements) is Humira. These drugs can reduce symptoms, but they come with a lot of side effects ranging from flu- and allergy-like aftereffects to a severe loss of blood pressure that can lead to death. They do not have regenerative properties. They do not cure your problem.

Importantly, they cost about $180,000 a year—which is partially covered by Medicare, Parts D and C (under Tier 5 in which you pay the highest percentage), and in rare cases, Part B. In fact, Medicare shelled out an estimated $4.7 billion in 2021 just for Humira alone.

All you readers who like jumping ahead know that last sentence is enough to trigger...

ONE LAST-WORD LIBERTARIAN RANT

I take the libertarian point of view regarding individual choices and responsibilities for personal health and life decisions. If, like those living on ocean fronts, though, you want to enjoy the good days and have all the rest of us pay for the reconstruction of your damaged home with our tax dollars—my answer is no.

Pay for your own choices. I have little respect for someone who knowingly spends a lifetime making poor food choices and then expects government-funded health insurance to fix the damage. However, if you want to build your home on a beach and it washes away every year, but you don't care because you take full financial responsibility when the storms come and you've got the money to rebuild it—well then, God bless. Likewise, if you want to eat sugar-filled donuts, fine—but don't break the health care system for the rest of us when you have a heart attack or other medical catastrophe because of your diet.

Let's look at the numbers. In May 2023, hedge fund mogul and billionaire Stanley Druckenmiller gave a keynote speech to graduating MBAs at the USC Marshall School of Business in which he described the impending health care/economic catastrophe.

During the 1960s, Medicare and Medicaid were lumped in with Social Security as part of our general entitlements program. Through those systems, we're currently spending 40% of our tax dollars on seniors. That expense represents *six* times the amount we spend on children. Keeping on this same path, that amount will become 60% in 20 years. In 25 years, it will be 70% of all tax revenue. The math is simple and obvious. The U.S. birth rate has dropped from a 3.7% postwar boom in 1957, to the current 2%. Young people are not having as many children as their grandparents and parents did. We don't have enough people paying enough taxes to support this cost trajectory.

I understand that demographics and economic policies may seem out of your individual control, but let's go back to that percentage of tax dollars currently being spent on seniors. I estimate that 80% goes toward the ever-soaring costs of health care for diseases caused by sugar. As a society and as individuals, we *all* are paying for every single case of sugar poisoning. Your first motivation to stop eating sugar is because it will improve your own health and longevity. Equally important, it will slow the velocity of tax revenues circling the drain into a financial abyss.

In his speech, Druckenmiller had no solution. I do.

Sugar causes the problem, and stem cells fix the problem. Meanwhile, if we continue denying these facts, we are dead—and so goes another great society. If we embrace the truth, we prosper and survive.

Bibliography

Adelson, Joel W., and Joanna K. Weinberg. "The California Stem Cell Initiative: Persuasion, Politics, and Public Science." *American Journal of Public Health* 100, no. 3 (2010): 446–451. https://doi.org/10.2105/AJPH.2009.168120.

Bojanic, Christine, Kendrick To, Bridget Zhang, and Christopher Mak. "Human Umbilical Cord Derived Mesenchymal Stem Cells in Peripheral Nerve Regeneration." *World Journal of Stem Cells* 12, no. 4 (2020): 288–302. https://dx.doi.org/10.4252/wjsc.v12.i4.288.

Cascio, Matthew A., and Taif Mukhdomi. "Small Fiber Neuropathy." StatPearls. Last updated December 12, 2022. https://www.ncbi.nlm.nih.gov/books/NBK582147.

Charitos, Ioannis Alexandros, Andrea Ballini, Stefania Cantore, Mariarosaria Boccellino, Marina Di Domenico, Elisa Borsani, Riccardo Nocini, Michele Di Cosola, Luigi Santacroce, and Lucrezia Bottalico. "Stem Cells: A Historical Review About Biological, Religious, and Ethical Issues." *Stem Cells International* (2001): 9978837. https://doi.org/10.1155/2021/9978837.

Cubanski, Juliette, and Tricia Neuman. "A Small Number of Drugs Account for a Large Share of Medicare Part D Spending." KFF. July 12, 2023. https://www.kff.org/medicare/issue-brief/a-small-number-of-drugs-account-for-a-large-share-of-medicare-part-d-spending/.

Druckenmiller, Stanley. "Stanley Druckenmiller | May 2023 | Keynote at USC Marshall." B2B Academy. Posted May 5, 2023. YouTube video, 1:06:41. https://www.youtube.com/watch?v=SRPMHinrFKQ.

Druckman, Michael N., Meredith Manning, and Ashley Grey. "O.K. Corral: FDA Sets Stage to Appeal California Stem Cell Treatment Center Decision." Hogan Lovells. January 19, 2023. https://www.engage.hoganlovells.com/knowledgeservices/news/ok-corral-fda-sets-stage-to-appeal-california-stem-cell-treatment-center-decision.

"Executive Order 13505: Removing Barriers to Responsible Scientific Research Involving Human Stem Cells." *Federal Register* 74, no. 46 (2009): 10667–10668. https://www.govinfo.gov/content/pkg/FR-2009-03-11/pdf/E9-5441.pdf.

Fiore, Kristina. "FDA Warns Company Over Amniotic Products." MedPage Today. July 27, 2023. https://www.medpagetoday.com/special-reports/features/105653.

Food and Drug Administration. "Human Cells, Tissues, and Cellular and Tissue-Based Products; Establishment Registration and Listing." *Federal Register* 66, no. 13 (2001): 21 CFR Parts 207, 807, and 1271. https://www.govinfo.gov/content/pkg/FR-2001-01-19/pdf/01-1126.pdf.

Gupta, Ashim, Saadiq F. El-Amin, Howard J. Levy, Rebecca Sze-Tu, Sobrasua E. Ibim, and Nicola Maffulli. "Umbilical Cord-Derived Wharton's Jelly for Regenerative Medicine Applications." *Journal of Orthopaedic Surgery and Research* 50, no. 1 (2020): 49, https://doi.org/10.1186/s13018-020-1553-7.

Jewett, Christina. "FDA's Drug Industry Fees Fuel Concerns Over Influence." *New York Times*, September 15, 2022. https://www.nytimes.com/2022/09/15/health/fda-drug-industry-fees.html.

Johnson, Stephen A., Kamal Shouman, Shahar Shelly, Paola Sandroni, Sarah E. Berini, P. James B. Dyck, Ernest Matthew Hoffman, Jay Mandrekar, Zhiyv Niu, Christopher J. Lamb,

Phillip A. Low, Wolfgang Singer, Michelle L. Mauermann, John Mills, Divyanshu Dubey, Nathan P. Staff, and Christopher J. Klein. "Small Fiber Neuropathy Incidence, Prevalence, Longitudinal Impairments, and Disability." *Neurology* 97, no. 22 (2021): e2236–e2247. https://doi.org/10.1212/WNL.0000000000012894.

"Leading Lobbying Industries in the United States in 2023, By Total Lobbying Spending." Statista. February 26, 2024. https://www.statista.com/statistics/257364/top-lobbying-industries-in-the-us.

"PRP Therapy vs. Stem Cell Therapy: What's the Difference?" Todd Peters MD. Accessed April 14, 2024. https://newportspinemd.com/prp-therapy-vs-stem-cell-therapy-whats-difference/.

"Regulatory Considerations for Human Cells, Tissues, and Cellular and Tissue-Based Products: Minimal Manipulation and Homologous Use." U.S. Department of Health and Human Services Food and Drug Administration. July 2020. https://www.fda.gov/media/109176/download.

James A. Thomson, Joseph Itskovitz-Eldor, Sander S. Shapiro, Michelle A. Waknitz, Jennifer J. Swiergiel, Vivienne S. Marshall, and Jeffrey M. Jones. "Embryonic Stem Cell Lines Derived from Human Blastocysts." *Science* 282, no. 5391 (1998):1145–1147. https://doi.org/10.1126/science.282.5391.1145.

United States v. US Stem Cell Clinic, LLC, No. 19-13276 (11th Cir. 2021). https://law.justia.com/cases/federal/appellate-courts/ca11/19-13381/19-13381-2021-06-02.html.

Walsh, Anne. K. "United States v. California Stem Cell Treatment Center." Food and Drug Law Institute. Accessed

April 14, 2024. https://www.fdli.org/2023/06/united-states-v-california-stem-cell-treatment-center/.

"Wicker Leads 94 Pro-Life Legislators in Call to End Taxpayer-Funded Embryonic Stem Cell Research." Roger Wicker U.S. Senator for Mississippi. September 4, 2020. https://www.wicker.senate.gov/2020/9/wicker-leads-94-pro-life-legislators-in-call-to-end-taxpayer-funded-embryonic-stem-cell-research.

CHAPTER 7

Un-*Glued* for Life

—*on becoming an urban carnivore*

Change is difficult—it takes patience and motivation. It's not enough to convince you to stop eating sugar without presenting reasonable, effective tools for practical, real-life change. Considering all the news reports and scientific studies about how the foods we eat affect disease, inflammation, pain, physical dysfunction, and even the acceleration of the symptoms of aging, why wouldn't most of us be confused about what to eat? Each new scientific food study contradicts the last. The "breakthrough" reports with headlines like "Science says eat this; never eat that," "These 10 foods fight cancer," "Watch out for these five foods that will probably kill you," appear at regular intervals. Which government agency, medical establishment, doctor, or pharmaceutical ad should you believe? What cures what, and what else just makes it itch more?

While greed and ineptitude in our food supply exists, most people are unaware of the overall consequences of everyday macro decisions. Who's to blame?

- The factory owner who pays employees to make sugar-crunchy treats, or the employer who lines the break room with vending machines stocked with poisons?
- The guy who backs the tanker full of grain (now full of sugar) up to the factory's loading dock, or the company that embeds prophylactic herbicides into seeds before the farmer even plants them in the ground?
- What about the farmer who must increase crop yield with undesirable methods if there's any hope of saving Grandpa's acreage?

Confusion is multiplied even by those charged with protecting us. Particularly in its advocacy of Big Agriculture and the production of grains, the USDA is either inept or a criminal organization—there's no doubt of it.[78]

Furthermore, dozens of organizations, such as the American Diabetes Association, have yet to recognize and advocate the mountain of scientific evidence that a low-carb/no-carb diet lowers blood-sugar levels, can decrease the need for artificial insulin, and prevents needless pain and suffering for tens of millions of Americans.

As a society, we need new food chain habits—new vigilance from our protectors. And while you, as an individual, have precious little chance of getting that accomplished, you *can* control what you pick

---

78 For one quick example, check out the FDA's conclusion that Frosted Flakes are healthier than an avocado: http://www.wsj.com/video/fda-frosted-flakes-healthier-than-an-avocado/7F1713E3-21F6-479F-8FEC-67B9365C9026.html.

up and put in your own mouth. Sugar tastes great—we all know that. And if there were a magic pill allowing us to eat sugar all day long, I'd probably take it too. But there is no such pill.

Still, there's always that hope of a shortcut.

Currently we're seeing a great deal of hype about a new class of "designer" glucose-controlling/weight-loss drugs that mimic the natural hormone GLP-1. Marketed under names such as Ozempic®, Wegovy®, Saxenda®, et al., these drugs come with a heavy dose of side effects, including muscle-mass loss,[79] diarrhea, nausea, constipation, and vomiting, which can lead to dehydration and severe kidney problems. Specifically, scientists have recorded in the *Journal of the American Medical Association* conditions such as gastroparesis, a highly consequential disorder that slows or stops the movement of food from the stomach to the intestine.

Instead, Big Pharma would rather you take a new semaglutide Ozempic-type drug, which gives you the ability to eat all you want because you've turned off the fat-storing gene. What's patently obvious is that you're also going to have to take said drug for the rest of your life. And if your lens is the corporate bottom line, great! Then they've gotcha. Enter more frustration because you're stuck even deeper—and must depend on these "scientists" to tell you what's right and what's wrong.

Moreover, the drugs are expensive. For example, the average cost of Ozempic® is $6.97 per daily injection, which averages $212 per month or $2,544 annually. There are generic forms of this drug,

---

79 Let us not forget that your internal organs such as heart, lungs, and stomach primarily consist of muscle tissue.

and they do tend to cost a bit less. The key point, however, is that if you don't change your eating habits, you will need to take such injections for the rest of your life—or the weight will return.

In the meantime, sugar is still killing you.

The work of Professor Thomas Seyfried, cancer biologist and researcher at Boston College, reaffirms that cancer cells feed almost exclusively on glucose. His conclusion verifies Otto Warburg's theory that cancer is a metabolic dysfunction wherein a cell's chief energy-producing mechanism—the mitochondria—goes into what Seyfried calls fermentation mode. In this state, the cell is unable to produce oxygen and can live only by the chemical process of fermentation—*a process driven by sugar.*

Ultimately, each of us must take charge of our own individual food choices.

THE COOKIE ON YOUR BACK

Still, there are days when you decide Häagen-Dazs˚ makes life bearable. You just can't let that happen every day or even every month. As discussed in chapter 3, refined sugars (especially HFCS) and processed carbohydrates are the most harmful ingredients you can introduce to the gut microbiome—to move onward into the nervous system, including your brain. Such knowledge is meaningless unless we can conquer an addiction to sugar and carbs and embrace the kind of high-protein, low-carbohydrate diet I advocate on my website, https://www.drjacoby.academy/courses/unglued. There, my simple message is that what you eat will either kill you or keep you well.

Beware—the picture isn't pretty. When I evaluate the relationships between modern disease and malady, I'm reminded of the film *Little Shop of Horrors*. It started as a '60s cult film (with Roger Corman and Jack Nicholson) and was adapted into an off-Broadway musical, which then became a rock/musical/horror/comedy film in the '80s. (That route is exactly how one scientific discovery leads to another, when you think about it.) The premise was simple. Seymour, a nebbish assistant florist, finds a talking plant and names her Audrey II, in honor of his coworker and woman of his dreams. As significant as the fact that the plant talked was how it also survived on human blood. The more vigorously the plant belts out her song, "Feed me, Seymour!" and the more Seymour complies, the more Audrey II ups the stakes. Will the talking/carnivorous plant take over the world? Or will Seymour and his true love save humankind? It's not unlike the battles we face with health, wellness, and the modern food chain.

Audrey II could obviously represent your addiction to carbohydrates (sugar, grains, or alcohol), but she could also be a metaphor for the greed and corruption of industrial food production in this country. Sometimes, it seems that as these societal/industrial/commercial forces seek higher profits, they're also using our guts as diabolical laboratories. Our nervous systems are the collateral damage.

We must first establish that sugar can be a true addiction—acknowledge that a "monster demanding constant attention" is real.

While the research regarding its addictive pattern is scant, it is not unlike food addiction. German clinical and biological psychologist Adrian Meule defines food addiction as consuming large amounts of a food for an extended period, engaging in repeated attempts to cut down, and continuing to eat this food despite adverse consequences. Dr. Nora Volkow, director of the National Institute on Drug Abuse, goes so far as to equate food addiction to the patterns seen in drug addiction—both of which present as dysfunction in the brain neurotransmitter, dopamine.

When feeding sugar water to rats, then periodically withdrawing and reintroducing the substance, Dr. Nichole Avena of Columbia University reported that the rats demonstrated distinct signs of addiction: binging, withdrawal, craving, and addiction transfer (i.e., addicts substituting caffeine for sugar or donuts for alcohol.) Just as in the *Little Shop of Horrors*, Audrey II gets progressively demanding when denied.

I have patients who insist that dessert signals them to stop eating a meal. They are unaware—or don't want to know—that salad with vinegar and oil does the same thing. So does a piece of fine cheese.

You can start with simple steps. Think of what's in your kitchen right now. How can you make simple changes for better health? If you can whip up cookies, a classic flan, or fudge from whatever ingredients you have on hand —get rid of them. The only exception may be if you make your own nectar for the hummingbird feeders.

Beyond what's in your pantry, other pitfalls hide in fairly plain sight—mainly in the picture of the product and the marketing words to attract you. "But," you say, "I read the package ingredients." The actual labels on processed foods can be deceiving, because while you may think the nutrition label on your box of crispy yummies is official, in truth, labels are created by the manufacturer. Any food start-up can make its own food nutrition label. Just check out www.recipal.com. It's all a matter of making a list and hiring a graphic designer.

Nevertheless, in large measure, you can still control what goes into your body. Even though most nuevo-health trends require you to pay more for locally grown, natural food, you can start making a change for health by growing even a single organic tomato in a patio pot or windowsill. Just buy organic seeds and plain garden soil, not those loaded with added chemical "benefits." Nor do you need a huge plot of land. Growing a variety of vegetables in small containers typically is enough for any family's meals. In addition, find ways to preserve them out of season.

EPIGENETICS AND GRANDMA'S TABLE

There are many healthy, natural diets and cuisines for you to model—and many more "experts" telling you *the* perfect one you must follow for optimal health. All this information is difficult to interpret, much less incorporate into your everyday life.

For example, a recent study making the media rounds purports that the Mediterranean diet, *when consumed with extra amounts of olive oil*, is linked to a reduction in the risk of breast cancer. Who wouldn't leap at such a promise? In covering the story, the prestigious Reuters explains the Spanish study and further reminds us of the general health benefits of the Mediterranean diet, which also replaces sugary desserts with fruit and nuts, favors fish over red meat, and limits beverages to mostly water and red wine. However, when you examine the original research, you find that it was supported by the California Walnut Commission, two Spanish

manufacturers of almonds and hazelnuts, the Spanish Ministry
of Agriculture, Fisheries and Food, and Fundación Patrimonio
Comunal Olivarero, a foundation and retail outlet dedicated to
the consumption of—you guessed it—olive oil.

THE KETOGENIC/PALEO CHOICE IS BETTER

My own study and research have led me to personally follow a
solid ketogenic (paleo) diet with abundant grass-fed animal protein and fat, reputably sourced fish and seafood, eggs, nuts and
seeds, full-fat dairy (cheese and cream, no milk), seasonal vegetables, and the occasional fresh fruit. Investigations from a team
at the Barrow Neurological Institute show that a ketogenic diet
reduces inflammation and swelling from fluids surrounding brain
tumors in mice. I'll take it.

Specifically, I advocate eating only grass-fed (sometimes called
grass-finished) proteins. Every dollar spent on currently high-
priced grass-fed protein is worth its biological weight in gold.
Contamination in factory farming—specifically, antibiotic-related
superbugs and general filth—will literally turn your stomach.

My first book editor once asked, "But what do *you yourself* eat?"

"I'm not a dietitian," I joked. "But my general rule of thumb is
that if it tastes good, don't eat it."

"Oh no," she replied. "We can't say that!"

The truth is that a high-protein/carnivore diet is delicious on its
most primal level. Once you substitute carbohydrates with protein,

your tastes change. Anyone ever placed on a highly restrictive low-salt diet knows that after a short while, rather than die, your taste buds adapt and don't even miss salt. And here's the secret: The same is true with sugar. Eliminating sugar full bore or cold turkey—or at least gradually—is the only tool available and the only one you'll need. It's a matter of self-responsibility. And once your taste buds have adapted, you'll see your desire for sugar subside, allowing you to severely limit it from your diet.

WHEN WILL WE EVER, FINALLY FORGIVE FAT?

Civilization celebrated many diverse accomplishments in the 1980s: the popularization of the cell phone, advancements of the MRI, the Rubik's cube, MTV, and the eradication of smallpox. However, "the no-fat, low-fat food fad" that peaked in this decade was not among them. Reinforcing inconclusive science that linked saturated (animal) fat to heart disease and cholesterol, the artificial-food industry used no-fat and low-fat labels as a marketing device to sell us more cookies, donuts, snack crackers, desserts, and breakfast cereals—crunchy treats of all kinds—made seductively hyperpalatable with high-fructose corn syrup (HFCS) and other refined sugars. Billions of dollars were made off countless products that implied these low-fat, high-sugar versions of your favorite foods could taste as good, be heart healthy, and still not make your jeans tight. Don't even get me started on Cheerios™— the "wonder cereal" once touted by superstars and now by Disney characters. However, these new products were made from an even more catastrophic chemical compound—partially hydrogenated oil, a key source of something called trans fat. That's when the fat game got very confusing.

Then in 2015, the USDA and Health and Human Services produced a scientific report from its Dietary Guidelines Advisory Committee tasked with updating information on which foods promote overall health.

The report eliminated warnings on dietary cholesterol. The panel determined that cholesterol "is *not* a nutrient of concern for overconsumption." In doing so, the Guidelines Committee reversed its earlier position that dietary cholesterol be limited to 300 mg (or roughly two eggs) per day.

Simply stated, eating saturated fat does not lead to high cholesterol. Human body fat is not made from animal fat. Rather, animal fat has a far more supreme function in the human biome.

In 2015, the *British Medical Journal* published a meta-analysis of 61 studies, involving more than 500,000 participants, which concluded that while higher intakes of saturated fat *were not* linked to mortality, coronary heart disease, ischemic stroke, or type 2 diabetes, consumption of unsaturated (or trans) fats *was* linked to significant increases in all-cause mortality and coronary heart disease due to the buildup of plaque inside the arteries.

The evidence was so conclusive that after the Dietary Guidelines Advisory Committee report of 2015, the FDA announced a ban of all partially hydrogenated oils (trans fat) in food—sort of. Variations are still found in these products:

- Commercial baked goods, such as cakes, cookies, and pies
- Shortening
- Microwave popcorn

- Frozen pizza
- Refrigerated dough, such as biscuits and rolls
- Fried foods, including french fries, donuts, and fried chicken
- Nondairy coffee creamer
- Margarine

Yet, many physicians are still stuck in past doctrines such as the cholesterol fraud. Physicians aren't the only ones who remain in the dark web of mistaken concepts, however. The cholesterol fraud still permeates our entire society. A recent trip to the grocery store brought me face-to-face with the results of that outdated scientific theory presented as gospel. The butcher had stripped all the health and flavor away, proudly presenting the assumed heart-saving favorites: boneless, skinless chicken breast and ground beef proudly declared *80%–90% lean*. The falsities of cholesterol have turned into a religious-like cult. And if you say anything to challenge doctrine—like Bruno[80]—you're declared a heretic.

After my spirited and unsuccessful discussion with the butcher about the benefits of animal fat, I was then completely frustrated by the grocery's compulsory self-checkout protocol. I entered the process with some trepidation but thought, "I'm trainable. I can do this."

It didn't work out that way. Granted, the machine *had* told me to weigh the bananas, but I didn't see the digital prompt; therefore, I didn't press the right button before the deadline with its ear-piercing buzzer.

---

80 In 1600, Giordano Bruno, then renowned Italian philosopher, was burned at the stake for declaring that Copernicus was wrong—the sun *does not* revolve around the earth, the universe *is* infinite, and other solar systems *do* exist. In other words, he got some thanks!

Of course, that infraction prompted the young clerk monitoring the scene to come over and say, "Just press the button."

"Okay," I say. "What button? The whole panel is filled with buttons."

"The one right in front of you," he yelled.

Amazingly, I was able to complete the task. The point is that if we can learn how to operate machines, why can't we learn how to "operate" our bodies? No one will monitor your health like you can, and few professionals are going to rush to your aid to instruct you.

EVOLUTION AND CULTURAL DIETS

As Earth's most prolific meat eater, we humans have evolved to digest much of the animal that comprised our primordial dinners—fat and all. And it's no coincidence that fat tastes delicious! The right level of marbling in a steak or sizzling bacon creates a savory sensation we are hardwired to crave.

The new science regarding cholesterol means that most of us need to reinfuse our diets with healthy animal fat. I'll speak to surviving vegetarianism later, but despite decades of research and billions of dollars, science has failed to establish a causal link between saturated fats and heart disease. Yet, most Americans still believe the brilliant marketing myths that corn flakes are better than bacon, and it's healthier if you strip the skin off a chicken breast.

I've developed a simple scale that helps you select healthy ketogenic fats by looking at proteins and oils through a simple color-coded lens.

GREEN—Go for it. Eat as much as you want of any fat product from animals that eat grass.

YELLOW—Eat in moderation. This category includes fat from a grain-fed animal.

RED—Do not eat trans-fatty acids (e.g., margarine or artificially produced hydrogenated oils).

Yet, I fully understand it doesn't suit everyone—for example **surviving vegetarianism**.

My vegetarian friends are quick to tell me they're healthy. And I believe them. I respect food choices based on animal rights and/ or the deplorable conditions of current food manufacturing. I also believe it takes some effort to obtain essential amino acids from plants alone, especially for growing children. The truth is that many vegetarians avoid meat and animal products to fill up instead on fruits, sugars, breads and pasta, foods deep fried in vegetable oil, and processed packages of soy products—none of which provides adequate protein for muscle and nerve health. And all of which (as well as the deadly processed sugars and starches hiding within their meatless alternatives) provide opportunity for concurrent gut-health problems and growth prospects for cancer cells.

THE FRENCH PARADOX—A VIABLE ALTERNATIVE

As for my patients who have difficulty with the full-bore paleo diet, I suggest a traditional French diet model—minus sugary desserts and, sadly, the bread. Why French? I do it for three simple reasons:

(1) something researchers call the French paradox, (2) the admirable cultural *attitude* with which the French approach food, and (3) when I want to splurge, it's my favorite. I could as easily present plans from Asian, Caribbean, or Scandinavian cuisines. For everyday life, it honestly doesn't matter much which natural path you choose if you simply and emphatically *cut out processed sugar and other starchy carbs*. If you can make that commitment at this very moment, then you can close the book and skip chapter 7. If not, read on.

The French paradox became a topic of great interest in the late 1980s when it was determined that France, with its culinary masterpieces, high consumption of saturated fat, and reputation for decadent pastries (eaten with restraint), had one of the world's lowest incidences of mortality from coronary heart disease.

Scientists have since challenged many of the early studies, unfortunately. Worse, the unfortunate influx of fast foods has brought the French—statistically speaking—more on par with the rest of the industrialized world. Nevertheless, as a culture, the French maintain their traditional outlook on food—they demand fresh, seasonal food; often skip breakfast; limit portions; practice intermittent fasting; and generally, don't snack.

Lunches in French schools are legendary. Students sit at tables set with ceramic dishes and cutlery, leisurely enjoy multicourse meals, and are then given an hour's recess to play off the calories.

French law even mandates that at least 50% of the food served in schools is organic and locally grown or prepared—many schools strive for 90% to 100%. As a result, the traditional French diet doesn't include as many carbohydrates as we might imagine (consuming an average 68.5 grams of sugar per day while Americans consume an average of 126.4 grams).

You don't need to move to France or *overthink making* a change in your food choices, but definitely make the change. Food should be simple. The typical time spent in line at a fast-food chain is more than it takes to buy and even cook a simple protein and/or some veggies. Instead, think of cooking as "reheating." It will taste better and be healthier. Concentrate on preparing and enjoying fresh food in the company of family or friends. Most importantly, take charge of what you eat, and you will immediately begin reversing the devastating effects of sugar poisoning.

THE FUTURE OF MEDICAL MONITORING

How do we integrate ourselves into the tech world as we age? This connection is a challenge to balance because of the conflict of dependency versus freedom. We know we must function as we age—that's a big deal. Yet take heart, as we're on the brink of remarkable change via medical intervention in the monitoring of our bodily functions, including metabolism and heart rate.

The first week in October 2023, I was asked to be the keynote speaker at a Med-Tech Convention. While there, I explored a company called MedWatch Technologies that produces a watch/monitor that will finally give you—the patient—independence by monitoring your glucose in real time, finally transcending that whole uncertainty about what and what not to eat. When the device reveals exactly what the food you're eating is specifically doing to your body, you don't need to go to a doctor for a prescription. You simply adjust the fuel you're putting into your body.

Another company called DexCom produces continuous glucose-
monitoring devices primarily for diabetes management. Sales are
robust because insurance companies like that a person can monitor glucose and thus avoid the catastrophes that can occur when
glucose spikes and plummets.

With these devices you can see how specific foods are affecting
your blood sugar level in real time. No more guesswork. The
new Med-Tech monitors not only can do that, but they also can
monitor all other bodily functions including metabolism. They
can predict diabetes long before prediabetes is a glimmer in your
family doc's eye. As discussed in chapter 3, that's exactly what
ADMA—the body's inflammatory measure—does.

Med-Tech's product is a noninvasive patch. It rests on the skin
and measures nanoparticles of light photons to determine how
your body is creating energy—metabolizing food—and does so by
determining the signature of molecules comprising the off-gases
of this process. You can monitor this continuous reading yourself
and see how one food or one portion size may or may not affect
your individual body chemistry. Think of it as your individual
epigenetics, displaying what you're eating and what it's doing to
you—personally, metabolically. This knowledge will once and for
all solve the vegan/carnivore dilemma for each of us.

Think about it. The feature not only means you can monitor
blood sugar without guessing or pricking into your bloodstream,
but you also can monitor *how each specific* food is making your
body store or burn fat, best oxygenate muscles (particularly the
heart), or open constricted veins, arteries, and nerves. For example, perhaps I eat an apple and my genes go wild, instantly raising

my blood sugar, whereas you eat an apple, and there's zero spike in blood sugar. The advancement is transformative because it helps eliminate the anxiety that those with metabolic disorders experience every day. With this device, you will lessen the chances of ending up with a doctor trying to sell you a drug. You control your food with the help of high tech.

These emerging companies are amazing. I've recently heard of a new one called Blink Technologies, which produces eyeglasses (matched with your prescription if you have one) with tiny cameras embedded in the frame. Put them on, and the cameras take a picture of your eye as you go about your daily routine. It analyzes the data and then predicts what eye disease might be developing— for example, macular degeneration, a disease primarily caused by sugar poisoning.

And imagine the implications for professional truckers as this technology can monitor eye movements and detect when a long-haul trucker might be falling asleep. Normally, these critical workers drive all night, pull into a truck stop, and load up on carbohydrates with their resulting sugar spikes, then insulin causes them to get drowsy, they doze off, and…

With these devices, we can bypass invasive tests like blood tests and monitor our own personal chemistries. That ability is of paramount importance as we try to live the life of the urban carnivore. It puts control back into the hands of the patient. No more need for arguments over specialized diets or *healthier* diets. You can employ the diet that is most healthy for you, rather than having the government and big-business mechanisms telling you to eat the food pyramid, or the Department of Agriculture's MyPlate graphic. And we know what happened with that little adventure. It has altered the health of millions of Americans and their progeny.

So, then, what is the future for doctors when we no longer need them to diagnose? Or more importantly perhaps: What is our future without those who misdiagnose? These new medical technologies speak directly to the real problem with the American medical system, because it's not there to help you change your behavior. Today, when you go to your doctor, they will check your blood pressure, determine if it's up a bit, and spring into action. They are there to write an Rx to immediately stop an uncomfortable or dangerous symptom, all of which allows you to continue the destructive behavior. Prescriptions are what doctors are trained to provide, and that's what the system rewards them for doing. That's all they're trained to do—and that's all they can do. You as the patient are stuck because you must depend upon them to interpret their language (of science) and tell you how to stay healthy.

Usually, however, they rely upon their measurements to guess what's really the cause of your high blood pressure. Still, they're apt to simply prescribe Lexapro[81] and send you out the door. Rarely do they take the time to learn that you may have come from the grocery store where you first unsuccessfully challenged the butcher and then failed "self-checkout" to boot.

It's frustrating because like that butcher, hard-working, frustrated doctors don't want to hear me or anybody else tell them the answer is for us to embrace our ancestorial carnivore or to stop

---

81 Used to treat depression and anxiety, Lexapro (escitalopram) is an antidepressant within the family of drugs known as selective serotonin reuptake inhibitors (SSRIs).

eating sugar, processed foods, and all the other poisons in our Big Farming, Big Pharma, Big Government food desert.

Meanwhile, most physicians are still stuck in past doctrines such as the cholesterol fraud. Who will finally declare it a fraud that still permeates our entire society and re-educate the medical profession? Among less than a handful of others, I stand alone.

The question remains: How do we integrate ourselves into the tech world as we age? We question and we research information electronically and more thoroughly so that we're not subject only to what is promoted by the government or pharmaceutical manufacturers and immediately declared truth through mainstream media. Moreover, we consider the firsthand knowledge and listen to opposing views of those who don't sit primarily on Capitol Hill. Remember also to tab past page 1 of your search results in your Google query.

Finally, I ask you to reconsider Earth's time frame. The creation of Earth's soil began in the Cambrian era, some 545–485 million years ago. In fewer than the five recent decades, we have poisoned its sources of good food and the nourishment its soil produces—making our food supply toxic and addictive.

The evolution of carnivores has brought you to the point of making vital food choices in the nanosecond that your single life represents. You would not be a sentient human surviving on plant matter alone if your primordial ancestors had done the same. Become informed!

Bibliography

"Adult Obesity Facts." Centers for Disease Control and
   Prevention. Last updated May 17, 2022. https://www.cdc.
   gov/obesity/data/adult.html.

Angell, Marcia. *The Truth About the Drug Companies: How They
   Deceive Us and What to Do About It.* New York: Random
   House, 2005.

Avena, Nicole. "The Food Addiction Model Is Appropriate for
   Use with Food." Presentation at The Food Forum Workshop
   on Relationships Between the Brain, Digestive System, and
   Eating Behavior. The National Institute of Medicine.

Canadian Agency for Drugs and Technologies in Health.
   "Pharmacoeconomic Review Report: Semaglutide
   (Ozempic): (Novo Nordisk Canada Inc.): Indication: For the
   Treatment of Adults Patients with Type 2 Diabetes Mellitus
   to Improve Glycemic Control, in Combination with
   Metformin (Second-Line Treatment), and in Combination
   with Metformin and Sulfonylurea (Third-Line Treatment)."
   National Library of Medicine. June 2019. https://www.ncbi.
   nlm.nih.gov/books/NBK543967.

de Sousa, Russell J., Andrew Mente, Adriana Maroleanu,
   Adrian I. Cozma, Vanessa Ha, Teruko Kishibe, Elizabeth
   Uleryk, Patrick Budylowski, Holger Schünemann, Joseph
   Beyene, and Sonia S Anand. "Intake of Saturated and Trans
   Unsaturated Fatty Acids and Risk of All-Cause Mortality,
   Cardiovascular Disease, and Type 2 Diabetes: Systematic
   Review and Meta-Analysis of Observational Studies." *BMJ*
   351 (2015): h3978. https://doi.org/10.1136/bmj.h3978.

DeJong, Colette, Thomas Aguillar, Chien-Wen Tseng, Grace
A. Lin, W. John Boscardin, and R. Adams Dudley.
"Pharmaceutical Industry-Sponsored Meals and Physicians
Prescribing Patterns for Medicare Beneficiaries." *JAMA
Internal Medicine* 176, no. 8 (2016): 1114–1122. https://
doi.org/10.1001/jamainternmed.2016.2765.

Dietary Guidelines Advisory Committee. "Scientific Report
of the 2015 Dietary Guidelines Advisory Committee:
Advisory Report to the Secretary of Health and Human
Services and the Secretary of Agriculture." U.S. Department
of Agriculture, Agricultural Research Service. February
2015. https://health.gov/sites/default/files/2019-09/
Scientific-Report-of-the-2015-Dietary-Guidelines-Advisory-
Committee.pdf.

Doyle, Kathryn. "Mediterranean Diet Plus Olive Oil May
Reduce Breast Cancer Risk." Reuters Health. September 14,
2015. www.reuters.com/article/2015/09/14/us-health-
oliveoil-breast-cancer-idUSKCNORE.

"Trans Fat." U.S. Food and Drug Administration. Last updated
August 30, 2023. https://www.fda.gov/food/food-additives-
petitions/trans-fat.

Hallberg, Sarah, and Osama Hamdy. "Before You Spend
$26,000 on Weight-Loss Surgery, Do This." *New York Times*,
September 10, 2016. https://www.nytimes.com/2016/09/11/
opinion/sunday/before-you-spend-26000-on-weight-loss-
surgery-do-this.html.

Hayward, Ed. "Targeting Cancer." July 2019. https://www.bc.
edu/bc-web/bcnews/science-tech-and-health/biology-and-
genetics/targeting-cancer.htmlhttps://www.bc.edu/bc-web/
bcnews/science-tech-and-health/biology-and-genetics/
targeting-cancer.html.

Lenharo, Mariana and *Nature*. "Popular Weight-Loss Drugs
   Come with Side Effects Recent Studies Evaluate Risks
   Associated with Drugs Such as Wegovy and Mounjaro."
   Scientific American, October 19, 2023. https://www.
   scientificamerican.com/article/popular-weight-loss-drugs-
   come-with-side-effects/.

Meule, Adrian. "How Prevalent Is 'Food Addiction'?" *Frontiers
   in Psychiatry* 2, no. 61 (2011). https://doi.org/10.3389/
   fpsyt.2011.00061.

Sorkin, Craig. "How Much Does Ozempic Cost Without
   Insurance?" K Health. September 8, 2022. https://khealth.
   com/learn/weight-loss/ozempic-cost-without-insurance.

"Statistics About Diabetes." American Diabetes Association.
   Accessed April 17, 2024. https://diabetes.org/about-diabetes/
   statistics/about-diabetes.

Stetka, Bret. "Fighting Cancer by Putting Tumor Cells on a Diet."
   NPR WNYC. March 5, 2016. https://www.npr.org/sections/
   health-shots/2016/03/05/468285545/fighting-cancer-by-
   putting-tumor-cells-on-a-diet.

Szalavitz, Maria. "Can Food Really Be Addictive? Yes, Says
   National Drug Expert." *Time*, April 05, 2012. https://
   healthland.time.com/2012/04/05/yes-food-can-be-addictive-
   says-the-director-of-the-national-institute-on-drug-abuse.

Taubes, Gary. *Why We Get Fat: And What to Do About It*, New
   York: Anchor Books, Random House, 2010.

Teicholz, Nina. *The Big Fat Surprise: Why Butter, Meat and Cheese
   Belong in a Healthy Diet*. New York: Simon and Schuster,
   2014.

"Trans Fats, But Not Saturated Fats, Linked to Death Risk."
   NewsMax. August 12, 2015. https://www.newsmax.com/

Health/Health-News/trans-fat-saturated-study/2015/08/12/
id/669708/.

Tinker, Ben. "Cholesterol in Food Not a Concern, New Report
Says." CNN. Last updated February 19, 2015. https://www.
cnn.com/2015/02/19/health/dietary-guidelines/index.html.

Toledo, Estefanía, Jordi Salas-Salvadó, Carolina Donat-Vargas,
Pilar Buil-Cosiales, Ramón Estruch, Emilio Ros, Dolores
Corella, Montserrat Fitó, Frank B. Hu, Fernando Arós,
Enrique Gómez-Gracia, Dora Romaguera, Manuel Ortega-
Calvo, Luís Serra-Majem, Xavier Pintó, Helmut Schröder,
Josep Basora, José Vicente Sorlí, Mònica Bulló, Merce Serra-
Mir, and Miguel A Martínez-González. "Mediterranean
Diet and Invasive Breast Cancer Risk Among Women
at High Cardiovascular Risk in the PEDIMED Trial: A
Randomized Clinical Trial." *JAMA Internal Medicine* 175,
no. 11 (2015): 1752–1760. https://doi.org/10.1001/
jamainternmed.2015.4838.

Epilogue

A few years ago, I attended a musical adaptation of Woody Allen's earlier film *Bullets Over Broadway*. Set in the raucous days of Prohibition, a struggling young playwright makes a simple mistake. He decides that the best way to finance his new play is to give a minor part to a mobster's ditzy, talentless girlfriend.

Soon, the girlfriend and the play's aging star squabble over who has the better lines. As the story evolves, the girlfriend's bodyguard suggests first one, then another line change to bolster her scenes. Gradually, the mob takes over the entire production, and the playwright can't recognize his own creation. I see this scenario as a metaphor for how Big Pharma has gradually taken over medicine.

Our nation faces an expanding health care crisis, and it's getting worse because Big Pharma runs the show. As discussed in chapter 6, the current rate of disease caused by sugar is breaking the medical system as the money we spend on health care (particularly through Medicaid and Medicare) far surpasses the amount scheduled to replenish the coffers of those social network programs.

This situation is an existential turning point not only for us as individuals, but for the financial health of the U.S. as well. I could say we're facing our own "bullets over medicine" catastrophe. That's a big claim, but I'm a student of history, and we find a similar situation if, for example, we look back to the Battle of the Nile and how the failure to correctly measure the incoming tide also led to the fall of a great nation. I argue the two events are the result of equally simple and cataclysmic mistakes.

In 1798, Napoleon sailed to Alexandria, Egypt, to establish a colony and thwart the British who had already gained a foothold in the rich African nation. Along with his troops, Napoleon deployed approximately 160 civilian scholars and scientists, known as the savants, many of whom were from the renowned Institut de France.

When news of the new French colony reached the British, they sent their own fleet commanded by Sir Horatio Nelson. Upon arrival at the mouth of the Nile, they discovered that somehow the French had miscalculated the tide and anchored too far out into Aboukir Bay. When the tide came in, that simple but deadly mistake allowed the British to cut between the shore and the French ships—and literally blow them out of the water.

Then in a magnificent twist of history and fate, the savants, stranded in Alexandria for the next 30 years, would be joined by other intellectuals to comprise the Institut d'Egypte. Left to lives of scientific observation and contemplation, this group of savants made momentous scientific observations regarding the precursory underpinnings of today's scientific accomplishments.

Two of their stories influenced me the most. Étienne Geoffroy Saint-Hilaire was a naturalist who came up with the unity of composition principle—a single consistent structural plan basic to all animals—meaning the basic anatomical similarities we share with other animals (mammals in particular). This premise became a major tenet of comparative anatomy and the division of animals into phyla. Saint-Hilaire also studied the eggs of various animals. When he tested them with different stimuli, he observed that a negative stimulus (a.k.a., trauma or stress) could change an animal's prodigy; thus, opening the door to the science of epigenetics and the idea that genetics are *not* immutable. That's a very big concept for the early 19th century.

Another savant survivor was Jean-Baptiste Joseph Fourier, the mathematician who started the chain of discovery leading to how we now launch and control satellites. His early work in the mathematics of light directly led to the creation of today's wearable health monitors. Engineers and scientists creating these devices are the savants of our nation.

At the risk of stretching the Woody Allen metaphor, we don't know all that's going on behind the health care scenery. But we do know that money will corrupt. And money does corrupt when you take out the eyeball-to-eyeball contact in any exchange. I personally think that deception is what really ails our 21st century world. It's not one government scheme or political party—Democrat or Republican. It's simply how the silent hand of commerce works—the nature of humans and economics. We would like somebody else (a.k.a., a government agency) to care for us.

"Give me all your money, and I'll see you in heaven."
That's the collective religious dogma.

"Give me all your money, and I'll take care of you in retirement." That's the Great Society.

"Give me all your money, and I'll make the pain stop." That's the promise from Big Pharma.

And they could be right—but at best it's a short-sighted plan, and at worst, an outright lie. I prefer Ronald Reagan's philosophy. When asked if he trusted America's Cold War adversaries, Reagan quipped the old Russian proverb: "Trust, but verify."

I hate to say it, but it's true. When you give control over your decisions to a third party, you get lazy, and you rely on that third party. Then, when they fail you, you're the one who suffers—while they sleep just fine at night.

Where Are We Now?

When my first book, *Sugar Crush*, was published, the solution seemed so simple to me—stop eating sugar so that I can stop amputating toes and legs. Case closed. Boy, was I wrong. Even though the evidence continues to mount, we still do not have universal recognition that sugar is causing hundreds of "-itises" and "-ectomies." I find it disgraceful and approaching criminal intent to add this poisoning of our diet and creation of disease. Worst of all, those in authority are slow-walking the cure.

A few months ago, I was asked to present at a medical meeting and once again, I pitched the same basic message and used the same slides that I'd created in 2011. I was right then, and I'm right now.

Also on the program was a radiologist from Stanford who gave a video presentation on MRI-PET scans along with an injectable tracer that allowed us to visualize everything thing I've been saying about the origins of disease. It's sugar. Period.

This new technology literally lights up an inflamed area, allowing physicians to watch as cells infused with magnetic nanoparticles actively target inflamed tumor cells in the brain left behind after surgical resection of the primary tumor. "Light it up; juice it up." It's that simple. One disease process...ten thousand areas of inflammation.

We now know what sugar does to our bodies. Any day of the week, I can scan the medical literature from across the globe and find new studies reaffirming foregone conclusions. As I write these final pages of *Un-Glued,* a quick online search reveals these results:

1. *Dietary Fructose Promotes Prostate Cancer Growth.*

Of course, it does. Otto Warburg got the Nobel Prize for proving it. Yet once again, researchers with Pontificia Universidad Católica de Chile demonstrated that fructose is a key metabolic substrate supporting prostate cancer cells, revealing potential therapeutic targets and biomarkers.

2. *Fructose Can Accelerate the Development of Breast Cancer.*

Scientists at the National Clinical Research Center for Cancer, Tianjin Medical University Cancer Institute and Hospital in Tianjin, China, report that "the fructose diet promoted metastasis of 4T1 cells in the mouse models. Our data...suggest that the high-fructose diet could accelerate the progress of breast cancer *in vivo.*[82] Furthermore, they conclude, "Fructose and glucose exert similar effects on proliferation and migration of cancer cells."

3. *High Sugar Consumption Is Linked to Alzheimer's Disease.*

In separate studies, researchers with both Wake Forrest University of Medicine and the Johns Hopkins University School of Medicine have linked elevated blood glucose and high levels of sugar intake with the development of the amyloid plaques found in the brains of individuals with Alzheimer's.

4. *It's Getting Worse.*

Researchers from the University of Texas conducted a meta-analysis of worldwide sugar consumption and increased cancer rates over a 45-year period. Specifically, the researchers tracked colorectal, breast, kidney, liver, pancreatic, uterine, and ovarian cancers—and what did they find? "Evidence from epidemiologic and preclinical studies demonstrates that excess sugar consumption can lead to development of cancer and progression of disease for those with cancer independent of the association between sugar and obesity."

The "proof" walks into my clinic every day. For example, I've been treating a patient's severe arthritis with stem cells, and last week he brought in his 28-year-old son who has severe Crohn's disease with fistulas (abnormal lesions) throughout the digestive system. Currently, the young man is being treated at the Mayo Clinic and is scheduled to have radical surgery to remove his colon. My patient and his son wanted to know if stem cells could help him. I

---

82 "In vivo" is simply Latin for a process taking place in living animals.

told them I couldn't help with the kinds of therapy he needed but that I could give him a referral to Riordan's clinic.

Then I asked, "What did the folks at Mayo tell you about diet?"

"We never discussed it," he answered.

Instead, they put him on Remicade—an immunosuppressive drug meant to control inflammation at $200,000 a year. And it hasn't worked. When we went over his diet, it was clear that he was a "sugarholic," and he had just burned out his gut. My recommendation was to immediately go to a carnivore diet and give that a chance before taking such a radical step of removing his colon.

Why are Big Pharma and Big Government slow-walking the cure? How can doctors at a world-premiere health institution remain unaware of the root cause? We need only return to the Upton Sinclair quote that opened chapter 4: "*It's difficult to get a man to understand something, when his salary depends on his not understanding it.*"

Perhaps it's better to ask "What can **you** do about it?" How can *you* beat the odds and outsmart the forces that are working against you? And in the greater scheme of things, can you outlast your retirement funds with this reliance on a failed medical system?

I've dedicated my career to sharing the important answers to such questions.

Sugar causes pain and disease. Stem cells can reverse the damage of a lifetime.

The choice—the responsibility—is yours.

Bibliography

Carreño, Daniela V., Néstor B. Corro, Javier F. Cerda-Infante, Carolina E. Echeverría, Catalina A. Asencio-Barría, Verónica A. Torres-Estay, Gonzalo A. Mayorga-Weber, Pablo A. Rojas, Loreto P. Véliz, Pedro A. Cisternas, Viviana P. Montecinos, Ignacio F. San Francisco, Manuel A. Varas-Godoy, Paula C. Sotomayor, Maite A. Castro, Francisco J. Nualart, Nibaldo C. Inestrosa, and Alejandro S. Godoy. "Dietary Fructose Promotes Prostate Cancer Growth." *Cancer Research* 81, no. 11 (2021): 2824–2834. https://doi.org/10.1158/0008-5472. CAN-19-0456.

Epner, Margeaux, Peiying Yang, Richard W. Wagner, and Lorenzo Cohen. "Understanding the Link Between Sugar and Cancer: An Examination of the Preclinical and Clinical Evidence." *Cancers (Basel)* 14, no. 24 (2022): 6042. https://doi.org/10.3390/cancers14246042.

Fan, Xiajing, Hongru Liu, Miao Liu, Yuanyuan Wang, Li Qiu, and Yanfen Cui. "Increased Utilization of Fructose Has a Positive Effect on the Development of Breast Cancer." *PeerJ* 5, 2017: e3804. https://doi.org/10.7717/peerj.3804.

"'Institut D'égypte' and the Description De L'égypte." Napoleon.org. Accessed April 16, 2024. https://www.napoleon.org/en/history-of-the-two-empires/articles/the-institut-degypte-and-the-description-de-legypte.

"Johns Hopkins Medicine Researchers Link Sugar-Studded Protein to Alzheimer's Disease." Johns Hopkins Medicine. May 25, 2022. https://www.hopkinsmedicine.org/news/newsroom/news-releases/2022/05/johns-hopkins-medicine-researchers-link-sugar-studded-protein-to-alzheimers-disease.

"PET/MRI in the Diagnosis of Chronic Pain." Stanford
Medicine Health Care. Accessed April 13, 2024. https://
stanfordhealthcare.org/trials/p/NCT03556137.html.

Wright, Myra. "Sweet Trouble: How Sugar Intake Might Increase
Alzheimer's Risk." Neuroscience News. May 22, 2023. https://
neurosciencenews.com/alzheimers-sugar-metabolism-23313/.

Wu, Meiying, Haixian Zhang, Changjun Tie, Chunhong Yan,
Zhiting Deng, Qian Wan, Xin Liu, Fei Yan, and Hairong
Zheng. "MR Imaging Tracking of Inflammation-Activatable
Engineered Neutrophils for Targeted Therapy of Surgically
Treated Glioma." *Nature Communications* 9, no. 1 (2018):
4777. https://doi.org/10.1038/s41467-018-07250-6.

Take Control of Your Health
Today

 Visit **rickjacoby.com** for more advice on how to get un-glued.

 Order special bulk purchases for your company, organization, or community at **rickjacoby.com**

 Book Dr. Jacoby for speaking and consultations via contact form at **rickjacoby.com**

CONNECT WITH DR. JACOBY AT...

- **Website:** rickjacoby.com
- **Facebook:** @Dr.RichardJacoby
- **LinkedIn:** Richard Jacoby, DPM
- **Youtube:** @jacobydpm

Thank you for reading!

Thank you for reading! If you enjoyed **Un-Glued**, please leave a review on Goodreads or on the retailer site where you purchased this book.

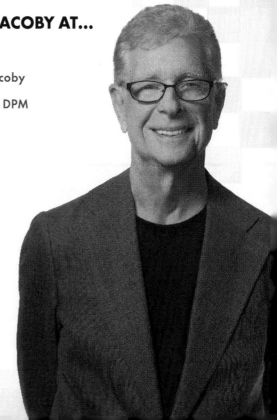

Made in United States
Orlando, FL
16 December 2024

55848057R00131